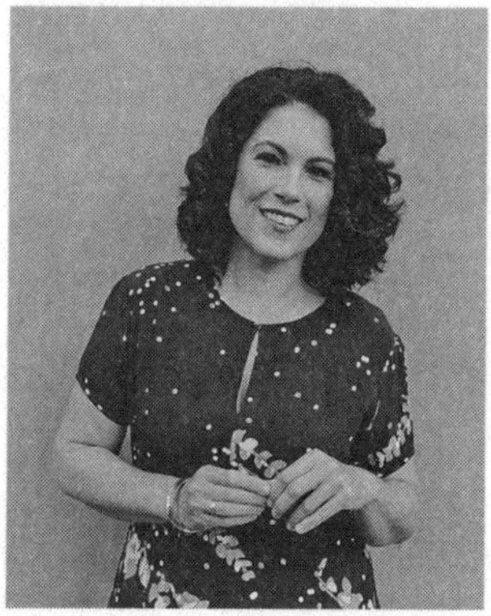

Rebecca Huntley is a writer and social researcher and a fellow of the Research Society of Australia. Rebecca was the director of The Mind & Mood Report and integral to developing the Climate Compass Project. She has also authored several books, including *How to Talk About Climate Change in a Way that Makes a Difference.*

SASSAFRAS

REBECCA HUNTLEY

hachette AUSTRALIA

Pseudonyms have been used in this book and other details altered to protect the identity and privacy of people mentioned.

hachette
AUSTRALIA

Published in Australia and New Zealand in 2024
by Hachette Australia
(an imprint of Hachette Australia Pty Limited)
Gadigal Country, Level 17, 207 Kent Street, Sydney, NSW 2000
www.hachette.com.au

Hachette Australia acknowledges and pays our respects to the past, present and future Traditional Owners and Custodians of Country throughout Australia and recognises the continuation of cultural, spiritual and educational practices of Aboriginal and Torres Strait Islander peoples. Our head office is located on the lands of the Gadigal people of the Eora Nation.

NATIONAL LIBRARY OF AUSTRALIA
A catalogue record for this book is available from the National Library of Australia

ISBN: 978 0 7336 5124 3 (paperback)

Cover design by Louisa Maggio
Cover image courtesy David Smart/iStock
Author photograph by Anna Turner
Typeset in 12.5/20 pt Bembo Std by Kirby Jones
Printed and bound in Australia by McPherson's Printing Group

FSC www.fsc.org MIX Paper from responsible sources FSC® C001695

The paper this book is printed on is certified against the Forest Stewardship Council® Standards. McPherson's Printing Group holds FSC® chain of custody certification SA-COC-005379. FSC® promotes environmentally responsible, socially beneficial and economically viable management of the world's forests.

Dedicated to my sister, Emily

And to 'Julia'

Give me truths,
For I am weary of the surfaces,
And die of inanition. If I knew
Only the herbs and simples of the wood,
Rue, cinquefoil, gill, vervain, and pimpernel,
Blue-vetch, and trillium, hawkweed, sassafras,
Milkweeds, and murky brakes, quaint pipes and sundew,
And rare and virtuous roots, which in these woods
Draw untold juices from the common earth,
Untold, unknown, and I could surely spell
Their fragrance, and their chemistry apply
By sweet affinities to human flesh
... Our eyes
Are armed, but we are strangers to the stars,
And strangers to the mystic beast and bird,
And strangers to the plant and to the mine;
The injured elements say, Not in us;
And night and day, ocean and continent,
Fire, plant, and mineral say, Not in us,
And haughtily return us stare for stare.
For we invade them impiously for gain,
We devastate them unreligiously,
And coldly ask their pottage, not their love.

Excerpt from *Blight* by Ralph Waldo Emerson, 1843

CONTENTS

AUTHOR'S NOTE

This book describes my experiences with MDMA as a therapeutic tool. I was fortunate to find a highly skilled and ethical practitioner who ensured these experiences were healing rather than damaging. I strongly support the ongoing, encouraging research on the role of MDMA for those managing trauma and PTSD. However, I am not a research scientist or medical doctor. Just because my experience was positive does not amount to an argument for the widespread use of MDMA. What was life-changing for me might be disastrous for another. This is powerful stuff that demands not only the right setting for its use but comprehensive care and ongoing support for the person taking it.

PART ONE

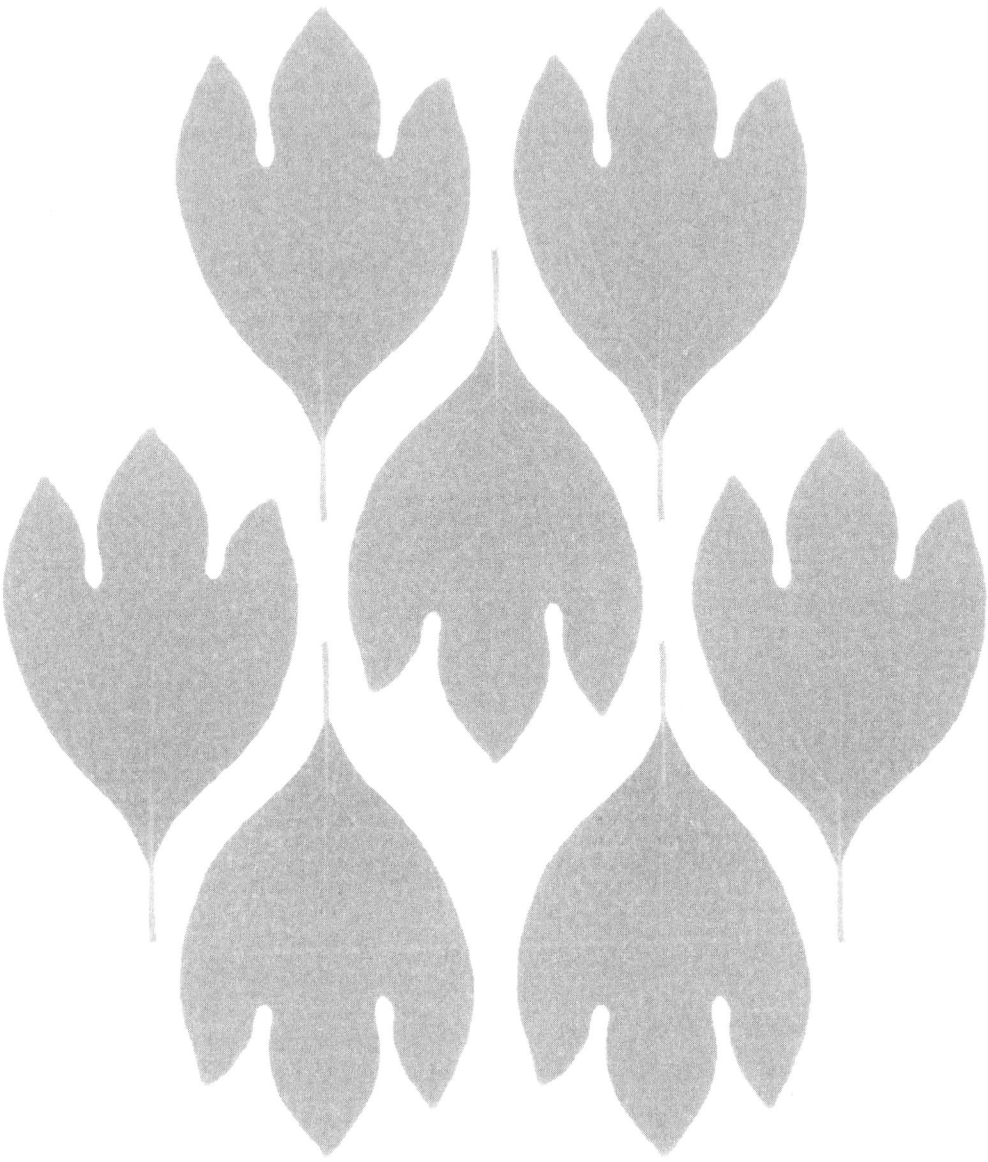

INTRODUCTION
Sassafras

I read about the sassafras tree long before I ever saw one.

That is not surprising. I was born in England, grew up in Australia and the sassafras is a ubiquitous American tree.

Also, I was not an outdoor child. I was the eldest daughter of a law professor and an English and History teacher, both happiest indoors with indoor pursuits. I was bookish and shy, not limber enough to climb a tree, even a modest one. Or brave enough to hike through woods.

Instead, I encountered the sassafras tree in the novels of Ntozake Shange and the poems of Walt Whitman and Ralph Waldo Emerson.

The sassafras is a fragrant, ornamental tree, with distinctive leaves that can look like a paw print. It grows at the forest's edge, as it needs some sun to thrive.

Europeans used the New World wood for shipbuilding and furniture making. Early toothbrushes were made from sassafras twigs, and the oil used as a dental anaesthetic, in soap, perfume and insect repellent. American settlers drank sassafras tea as a tonic. The Creoles used it to thicken soups. The British, who imported sassafras by the boatload, considered it 'lucky', capable of warding off evil spirits, and so they made protective objects out of it, inlays for cradles and boxes for bibles.

For Native Americans the natural oils in the wood and the leaves made it an excellent fire-starter. And it was used extensively to heal. The leaves, stems, bark and roots helped treat wounds, fevers, aches and pains.

The oil of the sassafras root, called safrole, can be used to make methylenedioxymethamphetamine, commonly known as MDMA.

I would have probably seen a sassafras tree when I was around ten years old, when I first travelled to Oregon and California with my parents and my sister. A family holiday wrapped around a work conference for my father. I remember how different the North American trees looked compared to the sparser casuarina and eucalyptus trees that grow along the coastline of Australia.

That miserable, confused child could never in a million years have guessed the virtuous root of this unfamiliar tree would one day help save her life.

*

Where do I begin?

My birth? The birth of any one of my children? The day my father walked out on us? The day I decided to stop speaking to my mother?

My first taste of MDMA at fifty years old on my living room couch?

In her book *The Art of Memoir*, Mary Karr says you should start with those memories 'you've nursed and worried over and talked through and wondered about your whole life'.[1]

Christ, there's a lot of them.

Some I have never forgotten. Others I re-remembered later in life, when the MDMA cracked me open and let those memories, good and bad, gush through the cracks.

Some of them I've never talked through except with my long-time therapist, and with myself inside my head. Over and again.

Before I can choose which 'nursed and worried' over memories to describe, I am wrestling with the problem of how much to describe.

How much truth do I need to tell in this story?

I could tell the whole story. Every horrible thing. What a drag a book like that would be. I pay my therapist well to listen to all that. One hundred and seventy-five dollars an hour. This book retails at a fifth of that price. So I'm giving you, the reader, the greatest hits.

Of course, there are the obligations to the living, the ones I love and the ones I don't want to hurt more than I already have. I am telling a story in which people, some very dear to me, are being cast against their will. I'm aware too, that I'm holding the pen and others in this story don't get that chance. I owe them something, those who can't write about what happened from their own perspective.

Those are my worries about the living.

The dead I don't really worry about. You can't defame them, and they already haunt me a little.

I'm scared, too. Scared this is going to end up like a 'wah-wah-white-girl' story, indulgent and self-pitying. And even though this is my second stab at memoir, I find writing about myself a hard task. It goes against all my training, in my early years as an academic and later as a social researcher. In my day job conducting interviews and focus groups, the questions are always directed towards others, the spotlight firmly on them.

In the past, when friends have suggested I write about my experiences with my parents, I've always recoiled. Why would I want to shine light into that darkness?

Looking back now, I realise it wasn't that my story wasn't worth telling; it was that I wasn't ready to tell it.

Then within a short period of time I got divorced, my father died, I cut ties with my mother, turned fifty, bought my first home of my own and did MDMA for the first time.

Then I was ready.

That being said, my story wouldn't be worth the paper it's printed on if it didn't lead to something bigger than what happened to me. Towards a larger story about what I have discovered about healing, about community and connection, about motherhood, about love and friendship in a time of climate crisis.

Mary Karr says, 'start with a memory you'd swear by'.[2]

This is it.

Chocolate cake for Christmas

The room was dark except for the light that penetrated in slivers around the drawn blinds. It was a sunny, hot afternoon a week before Christmas in my home town of Adelaide. I was about eight years old. I sat on a chair in the middle of the bedroom I shared with my younger sister, who was somewhere in the house. Hiding, probably. Understandably.

My mother stood by the door. In the dim light, I couldn't make out the expression on her face, but I didn't look to her for concern or pity. Or love.

I was focused on my father, who entered the room, fuming, carrying a chocolate cake, which he placed on a low table in front of me.

'You want to eat? Well, eat. You are going to eat all of this chocolate cake. Right now.'

I was, without a doubt, an unhappy child. Glasses, frizzy hair. Chubby and getting chubbier. Defiant. A daily provocation for my father, who had also been a chubby child with glasses. An embarrassment to my mother who was taunted by her father about her weight most of her adult life.

A few hours before, we had been visiting neighbours for a Christmas tea party. After we'd all eaten, the children had been dismissed to one of the bedrooms to play. The parents stayed sitting in the lounge room with the spread of food. I had walked back in, hoping to have some more.

I could always eat more. Even when I was full, I wanted more.

As I entered the room, my father looked up at me and said loudly, 'I think that's enough food for *you*, Rebecca.' I stomped out, hotly angry. I had left the lounge room door ajar, however, which meant the adults heard me say to the other kids, 'Sometimes I really hate my father.'

I had shamed him, and he was enraged. His need to be loved and obeyed without question was obvious to me even at that age. He was angry too that I was clearly failing to be a thin, fetching, 'easy' child. Or maybe he was just angry because I reminded him of him.

As we walked home soon after, I knew something was

very wrong, even before my mother whispered, 'He heard what you said.'

Of course, even as a baby I was a determined character, or so my mother used to tell me on a regular basis. I looked at the chocolate cake and then up at my father and thought, *I can do this.*

As chocolate cakes go, it wasn't that intimidating. It was one of those small, un-iced, chocolate sponges you get at the supermarket. Maybe something Mum was planning to decorate later with whipped cream and strawberries for Christmas guests.

I ate. One slice. Two. Then three. He stood over me as I ate. I began to feel sick. I said weakly, 'I can't eat any more.'

'You will eat it. The whole thing.'

'I can't.'

He put one hand firmly around the base of my neck so I couldn't pull away and started to shove handfuls of chocolate cake into my mouth.

'You will eat it.'

I started to gag, then to vomit, the fresh chocolate cake coming up first, and then what I'd eaten at the neighbours' house earlier. The vomit came up and out through my nose and my mouth, around his hands and down my neck.

I struggled to breathe through the vomit and his fingers in my mouth. Then it stopped. Maybe he stopped.

Maybe my mother made him stop. She would always intervene. Eventually.

I recall her leading me out of my room, down the corridor and through the kitchen into the bathroom. She helped me take off my spoiled clothes and guided me into the shower, where I washed off the vomit and tears and sweat.

She wrapped me in a towel and I sat on the bathroom floor, leaning against the toilet, soothed a little by the cool feeling of the cistern on my back and the tiles under my feet.

She left and returned with a wrapped Christmas gift, one she'd retrieved from under our plastic tree. I opened it. It was a new nightgown, white with little flowers. She put it on me. She seemed calm, rather than annoyed that I had provoked my father. The early Christmas gift I interpreted as some kind of admission that what had just happened required some restitution. I wondered if she felt sorry for me.

She told me what she often said when these things happened. 'You can't upset your father. He's very stressed about work. You need to remember: he is the child, so you need to be the grown-up.'

This wasn't the first or the last time my father exploded with rage at me. Not the first or the last time my mother stood by and watched it happen.

This is the memory I swear by.

It wasn't until I was in my mid-teens, sitting on my mother's bed, speaking about my father, by then long gone, that I remembered the story. I'd forgotten it and then – to use a cliché, because it's so accurate it seems silly not to – the memory came flooding back.

'That happened, didn't it?' I asked her. She nodded but didn't say anything.

Had I looked to her for a sign of concern, pity, love? Guilt and shame?

I can't remember.

*

That's one place to start. The technicolour memory that stands out against the greyish blur of everyday childhood comings and goings.

I start with the grotesque and the humiliating to prove that I mean business. But I promise I won't tell you more than you can handle.

There is another, probably better, place to start. Less upsetting, more recent, but just as significant.

Unlike the fragmented stories of my childhood, this is a series of events that lends itself better to a story you can follow. It starts with turning fifty, way past the halfway mark of my life. Still standing after a series of heavy emotional blows and big life changes – fertility problems, death and divorce under the pall of the pandemic, moving house more times than I'd care to remember, and realising that all the tools I'd used for years to block out the pain and anger weren't working anymore.

But first, some backstory.

1373 kilometres from Adelaide to Sydney

I was born in Oxford, England, but Adelaide was my first home town. It's a small city, nestled on the coast and surrounded by hills and ranges. It was established by wealthy free colonists who built a lot of churches and planted a lot of grapevines. It's missing the edgy convict past of my second home town, Sydney.

I grew up in a suburb near the sea, Glenelg North, where the state of South Australia was first proclaimed by white colonists at The Old Gum Tree in 1836. For a while, my mother's parents – Italian migrants who'd arrived in Australia before the Second World War – lived next door to this bent eucalyptus. My sister and I would play under and around it when we'd come to visit them, running our hands over its strangely curving trunk.

We – my mother, my father, my sister and I – lived in an elegant bluestone cottage spitting distance from the dank

Patawalonga River and walking distance from Glenelg Beach. Usefully close to Nonna and Nonno, who were always around, always helping. My younger sister spent so much time with them as a preschooler she was practically bilingual.

My earliest memory is of running barefoot around the perimeter of our cottage on a summer's day. Across the wide verandah with its tessellated tiles, then left, down the narrow passage between our house and our neighbour's, feeling the mixture of weeds, grass and pebbles under my feet. Across our yard with its clothes line and plastic paddling pool and concrete slab carport, then left again, down the other side of the house, this passage not as narrow, and paved with bricks. I remember slowing down along this passage, tiptoeing so as not to make a sound as I passed a window with the blinds always drawn. This was my father's study. And then, once I was certain I hadn't disturbed him in any way, accelerating towards my starting point in the front garden.

My second-earliest memory is of running away. I couldn't have been more than six, and I can't remember the incident that triggered it. I remember feeling angry about something my parents had done and deciding that running away was the solution. I had a brown, rectangular schoolbag, the kind made of reinforced cardboard with clips that would open with a loud click. I put a toy, a few silver coins and a book inside. I considered going into the kitchen to get some food but didn't – a clear oversight on my part, as I'd discover later.

I put on my sandals and walked out the back door, across the yard, out the wooden gate and along the laneway behind our house. When I reached the street, I began to feel less determined and more anxious. It was the furthest I had ever been from home by myself. I persevered, walking bag in hand down the familiar street that led past my best friend Lisa's house, towards what I felt would be good alternative housing for me: the covered part of the slippery dip at the local playground.

When I reached the playground there was no-one around. It was practically deserted. I climbed the stairs to the little alcove at the top of the slide, sat down, opened my bag and took out my book. I tried to read the pages of my Little Golden Book, but I couldn't concentrate. I looked at the coins at the bottom of my bag – they seemed entirely pathetic outside of the piggy bank in my room. I felt hungry in anticipation of dinner time, which was not far away. Why hadn't I stopped on my way out of the house to grab some fruit? I wondered if my mother might be worried about me.

Beginning to doubt the wisdom of my plan, I made my way back down the slippery-dip stairs and ran-walked my way back along the route I had taken, almost sprinting through the wooden gate and into the house.

No-one had noticed I'd been gone.

Dad was still locked in his study, my sister in the lounge room with her toys, my mother in her bedroom.

At least I didn't get into trouble, I told myself as I pushed my still-packed bag under my bed, ready for the next time.

Decades after this failed escape, I was with my eldest daughter, cleaning up her room. She was about five years old and we were sorting through broken toys and ripped clothes, working out what could be mended or donated. I started pulling out items from beneath her bed – odd socks, Lego pieces, rubbish, empty glasses, all the detritus that gets trapped under kids' furniture.

'Where's your running-away bag?' I asked her.

She looked at me blankly.

'What?'

'You know, the bag you keep under your bed for when you run away. Where is it?'

I realised it had never occurred to her that she might need such a bag. I felt an enormous sense of relief and satisfaction, but also a flicker of sadness for my younger self and her sorry little bag full of coins.

Despite it all, Adelaide had its comforting routines. We'd swim at the beach under the watchful eye of my Italian grandparents. We'd hang out with my nonna in her kitchen while she cooked one delicious dish after another – gnocchi, zucchini flower fritters, crostoli and lasagne. Sometimes we'd visit my nonno in his extensive garden and dusty shed.

My parents hosted elegant dinner parties where my mother would wear lipstick and my father would be jovial. He loved to entertain almost as much as my mother disliked cooking for other people. I'd wake up the next morning before everyone else and creep into the lounge room to eat the mint chocolates that hadn't been consumed the night before.

We had a black cat called Baffi, except we called her Buffy. Baffi is the Italian word for 'moustache', and Mum used to make us laugh by holding her wiggling tail under her nose and making a funny face. Looking back, I can see she was trying to bring some lightness into our heavy home, especially when Dad wasn't there. She'd play songs on our upright piano and my sister and I would dance around the coffee table. She'd hide a Bee Gees album under the record player, because Dad hated pop music. When he'd leave for work on the weekends, she would pull it out and play 'Staying Alive' on the turntable and we'd all dance.

And while Dad worked every day for hours on end, he'd read to us at night before bed. Poems, mainly – Ogden Nash and AA Milne.

What is the matter with Mary-Jane?
She's perfectly well and she hasn't a pain.
And it's lovely rice pudding for dinner. Again.

He loved that poem. He laughed after reciting it every time, and I knew the lines by heart. The cause of Mary-Jane's distress was obvious to any adult who cared enough to pay attention. After reading to us he would give us 'mad kisses', a flurry of kisses all over our cheeks and neck that would make us writhe and giggle.

There were bedtime poems and mad kisses, and there were also Sunday walks. After spending the day in his study, Dad would walk my sister and me across the park, towards the old-fashioned carousel by the sea. If we were well behaved, we'd get one ride on the white and black horses with real horsehair manes, then we'd have ice cream. I'd pick a white horse, and lemon gelato in a cup.

These are the sunny moments scattered throughout a childhood of walking on eggshells. I always knew that, no matter what, violence was coming. You could feel the tension growing, my father getting more frustrated, more short-tempered as the days passed. And then I would do something. Leave a wet towel on the floor. Eat the last chocolate chip biscuit. Say something wrong in front of the neighbours. *Kaboom*.

The violence felt inevitable but, perversely, it also felt like it was my fault. Like my lack of discipline, my selfishness had caused Dad to erupt. Afterwards there would be a few days, sometimes even a week, where things would be quiet and

I would be left in peace with my shame. Then the tension would begin to mount again, and the cycle would repeat itself.

Sometimes I would read books or watch TV shows where children knowingly did something wrong, broke a particular rule their parents had clearly articulated, and were punished in a ritualistic kind of way. Smacks on the bottom or slaps over the hand with a wooden spoon. I would absorb these stories, bemused. I'd have little sympathy for the children gritting their teeth through the pain or rubbing their welts afterwards with tears streaming down their faces. They knew the rules and they broke them. Idiots.

While I knew the violence would come, I never knew exactly what would set it off. There were no rules. Like I said, you could feel the tension grow as my father became increasingly stressed with work. He was in his late twenties and at the beginning of his brilliant career. He had an insatiable need to be feted and promoted. Any apparent bump in the road towards his goal – to be the greatest international lawyer in the world – would make him wild with frustration.

On days when something happened at work, even something minor, that threatened to thwart his progress – perhaps he had an article rejected by a journal, or was overlooked for a certain committee – he would come home fit to burst. And then he might walk into my room and see something that upset him. *Kaboom.*

One time as I was getting dressed after my evening bath, he was walking past my doorway and saw me tucking my white cotton singlet into my underpants in a way he found objectionable. He ran over, grabbed me by the arms and lifted me up so I was level with his sweaty, enraged face and started to shake me. '*Why are you doing that stupid, stupid thing?*' he yelled into my face, and shook me for what seemed like a minute but might have been less than ten seconds. When he finally released me, I dropped to the floor in a heap.

I think that's why I don't like rollercoasters.

Mum was capable of rages too, but not with the same frequency as my father. She was the more loving, more present parent and we clung to her. I idolised her. She was beautiful and funny and clever, and when she was in the mood, she could be joyful. But she could also explode like my father in unexpected ways.

On my seventh birthday I woke to find my gifts on the end of my bed, as was our family tradition. I had a much-treasured doll's house at the time, and Christmas and birthdays were a chance to furnish it. Ripping open the wrapping paper I discovered a tiny bookcase with tiny little books. The little books were glued shut, and I worked them open with my fingers so I could see the blank pages inside. I ran to my parents, who were still in bed, and showed my mother the little books.

'Where did you get those, Rebecca?' my mother asked.

'I made them.' It was a lie, and even at the time I wasn't sure why I said it. I was still thinking about the satisfying feeling of liberating the little pages from the glue.

I suddenly felt the full force of my mother's open hand across my cheek.

'You are lying,' she screamed at me. 'That's a lie. I bought those for you.'

My eyes filling with tears and my cheek stinging, I stood motionless, filled with shame that I had ruined my own birthday.

*

When I turned fifty, I walked the Camino de Santiago through northern Spain.

Don't be too impressed. I didn't walk all of it, and I walked it in luxurious conditions, as part of a small tour of wealthy Americans supported by two young Spanish guides who fed and watered us at every turn. We stayed in medieval palaces and ate at great restaurants.

This bookish, not-outdoorsy child who wouldn't climb trees or walk through forests had, by the time she was fifty, become a hiker.

I fell in love with walking when my first love broke up with me at twenty. I walked and walked around the streets of my suburb to get over the shock and the heartache. Heartache made worse by the fact that I knew I had been horrible to him, and that his decision had been the right one.

I was a long-haul city walker until I discovered multi-day bush hiking in my early thirties. Regardless of the terrain, for the last thirty years walking has been my tonic. It makes me feel both calm and strong, and provides the kind of release and blissful exhaustion I've never felt outside of sex.

Over the years, I've realised how important walking has been to my intellectual life. I've paced my way through work problems and blocks in my writing, unlocked ideas for new work and discovered new ways of thinking about the world.

In her book *Wanderers*, Kerri Andrews describes walking as 'soothing and useful',[3] and for decades that's exactly what it was for me.

Somewhere in my mid-thirties, I decided I would walk the Camino when I was fifty.

The Camino is an ancient pilgrimage route where, according to Catholic lore, all sins can be forgiven. Non-believers walk the route in pursuit of more secular enlightenment, that endless search for meaning and purpose. I wasn't searching for meaning and purpose, just peace and the chance to experience Spain, a country I'd never visited before, in a slow, immersive way.

A few weeks after my fiftieth birthday, I headed off for the 'highlights' version of this famous walk, expecting to experience the same kind of calm I'd found on my Australian hikes, only with tapas.

But instead of finding peace, I found myself tramping through the Galician scenery, along dirt-packed roads through villages, up rocky mountain sides, through cobblestoned alleyways and terraced vineyards with my mind churning through scenes of my childhood. My father, my mother, my father, my mother. Memories of them together, then apart, then together again. A memory-laden whirligig that never really stopped spinning, even when I was sleeping.

Along the Camino trail, waymarkers with a distinctive yellow shell count down the distance to your destination, like a medieval GPS. The town of Santiago de Compostela, the home of the shrine of St James the Great, is where most pilgrims end their journey. But the zero waymarker is located about an hour or so drive away from Santiago de Compostela, in the little seaside town of Fisterra.

Our band of *pellegrinos* made our way up the coast to the Fisterra lighthouse on a clear and sunny day, with me powering ahead. While my American pals poked around and took photos, I lay down on a stone bench, looking up at the sky, hugging my knees to my chest. It was 'the end of the world', and of my walk, and yet the whirligig was still turning.

Suddenly, a face loomed into view. Jack from California was looking down at me.

'Sore back huh, Aussie girl?' He spoke with the kind of drawl I associate with heroes wearing big hats in black and white films.

I sat up quickly. Jack had been one of the only Americans on the trip who I hadn't talked to much. I suspected he voted for Trump based on his chitchat over lunches, so I kept my distance. He'd done the same, so it was a surprise he was keen to talk to me now, so close to the end of our six-day tour.

'Just a bit of a stretch in the sun,' I said with a smile.

'You know, Aussie girl, I've been watching you on this trip and you know what I've worked out?'

'No, what have you worked out?'

'I reckon, if you wanted to, you could beat the crap out of me.'

I laughed and said I wasn't sure if that was a compliment or not. He went on to tell me I wouldn't have been able to 'bring him down when he was in his prime', and that his father was at Normandy.

I listened politely, if somewhat distractedly.

My immediate thought had been, *I sure could beat the crap out of you, just give me a chance.*

There was so much anger inside me. At the end of this long walk through Spain, my anger was so intense I felt that if it could take solid form, it could firebomb houses, level office buildings, blast through walls.

The next day, I said goodbye to the guides and the Americans on a rainy morning in front of the Cathedral in Santiago, wondering if I would ever be free of this endless rage.

Wondering – worrying – that maybe walking wasn't working for me anymore.

*

I was still feeling uneasy as I flew from Santiago to Madrid for the last few days of my holiday.

I was meeting up with my friend Kate, who had made the trip from Ireland to Spain to spend a few days with me. She asked if a Sydney-based friend of hers could join us, and I agreed. Nicky is a clinical psychologist. She has that grounded wisdom, that calm and attentive listening style all the best therapists have. The three of us wandered around food markets and drank spritzes on the top of buildings and gawped at *Guernica*.

On our last night together, we ate dinner at a bistro close to our hotel. As we waited for our food to arrive, Nicky wondered aloud whether she should call her mother back in Sydney for her birthday. It was a complicated relationship, she said, and she shared some of their story with me.

Over dinner, the three of us talked about the complexities of mother/daughter relationships. Eventually, Nicky shifted her focus from her dinner plate towards me.

'Kate has told me a bit about what's happening with you at the moment, with your mother.'

She took out a piece of paper and started writing down some book titles.

'I want you to go home and read these.'

I looked at the paper. Bessel van der Kolk's *The Body Keeps the Score: Brain, Mind, and Body in the Healing of Trauma* and Bruce D Perry and Oprah Winfrey, *What Happened to You? Conversations on Trauma, Resilience, and Healing.*

'*What Happened to You?* is an easy read. Start with that,' Nicky said. 'And *The Body Keeps the Score* is a classic text in trauma studies.'

I took the list and thought to myself, *Trauma? Is that what I'm dealing with here?*

I had never attached the word 'trauma' to what I had experienced as a child. If I was asked to describe my childhood, I would have said it was unhappy. Dysfunctional. Full of conflict. But not traumatic. That was a term for war veterans, foster kids and girls who had been raped by relatives.

My house is full of books friends have pressed into my hands that I have carried with me for years, their spines still pristine. But when I went back to my hotel room after dinner that night, something made me order those books online.

Maybe I was searching for new answers to soothe me, now that walking wasn't working quite so well.

The books arrived at my home a few days after I did, and on my first quiet weekend, I started reading.

*

I wolfed the books down in a matter of days, pausing only for toilet breaks, food and sleep. I would read a few pages and then close my eyes to let a revelation sink in. It was as if I had found a user manual for my own dysfunction and that of my family.

While both books had a profound impact on me, *What Happened to You?* is the one I read first, as Nicky had recommended, and it's the one I keep coming back to. Oprah needs no introduction ('*You have trauma, and you have trauma, and you have trauma!*'). Her co-author, Dr Bruce Perry, is a child psychiatrist and neuroscientist with a history of working with veterans and abused children. He was a regular on her show. The book is a transcript of them in conversation, punctuated by stories of her life and case studies from his practice.

The book helped me understand how trauma affects the brain. I knew about the 'fight or flight' response, but was largely ignorant about the ways ongoing stress, particularly during childhood, impacts the way the brain works.

Early in the book Perry explains that the brain is organised in a hierarchical way. The first layer is the brain stem, sometimes referred to as 'the lizard brain', which is responsible for primitive survival instincts and basic bodily functions. Next is the diencephalon, responsible for sleep and appetite. I knew a little about the limbic system, associated with reward, memory, bonding and emotions, so important to the relationship between parent and child from birth onwards. That's where the amygdala sits, a small, almond-shaped structure that's key to how we process strong emotions like fear, and how we tie emotional meanings to our memories. And then, finally, there's the higher brain, the cortex, the most sophisticated part of the brain, associated with thinking, language and reason.

When a person experiences any stimulus – vision, hearing, touch, smell – that stimulus is 'funnelled' through the four layers, starting with the lizard brain. 'Once the signal comes into the brain stem, it is processed … and matched against any previously stored experiences,' Perry explains.[4]

If those previously stored experiences are traumatic, even if you don't remember them, the brain stem can take over and register this stimulus as a threat, affecting all the following brain functions.

That's why vision, hearing, touch or smell connected to a traumatic event can trigger a full-blown stress response in someone who hasn't adequately addressed that underlying trauma.

It's why people who have PTSD from combat dread fireworks. Why children who have been abused by someone react badly to another adult who wears the same aftershave as their abuser.

As I worked my way through *What Happened to You?* I ticked off all the evidence of early childhood trauma manifest in my habits, quirks and worst impulses.

If I'm alone in a room and someone suddenly walks in, particularly if it's a man, even if I already know they're in the house, I startle and scream. I hate surprise parties. I've got no problem with spoilers – I google the end of every book I start reading or movie I start watching because I can't stand the tension of not knowing what's going to happen. I instinctively sit with my back against the wall in restaurants or meeting rooms so I can see who's coming towards me.

I realised, too, that the traits I like most about myself, the things that attract approval and accolades and are part and parcel of my 'success', are also a consequence of unaddressed trauma. When I am upset, I clean frantically. I have a near-spotless home. When I feel alone, isolated, I throw myself into my work. I am just shy of being a workaholic, that impulse tempered only by my love for my children and my friends. I throw myself into relationships, to the brink of exhaustion, always worried I'm not giving enough.

Unaddressed trauma drives my most shameful behaviour as well. I have an explosive temper. I have thrown bowls of food. Glasses and other hard objects, like telephones. I've hurled cakes into the sink, tipped a television onto the floor and taken scissors to clothing. I've slapped people. And I have written many, many angry emails – and sent them.

Perry's book revealed all my admirable, strange and destructive behaviour to be a stress response to unaddressed trauma. On the plus side, it also showed me I was already doing all the 'healthy' things that soothe the stress response, those regulating activities that balance out the food-throwing impulses. Walking in nature. Meaningful work. Healthy friendships. And therapy.

So much fucking therapy.

So, what's wrong with me?

I had read the books Nicky had suggested out of curiosity, but without high expectations. What more could I possibly learn about myself that at fifty, after thirty years of therapy, I didn't already know?

Therapy has paid off for me, despite a false start at fifteen. Dad was gone, the divorce was finalised and Mum thought she should seek the advice of a shrink. She thought I needed to see one too.

She booked us back-to-back sessions with an older man in a suburb close by. 'Close by' was the main requirement – she didn't want to drive far. Mum went first, while I sat flicking through magazines in the waiting room. When she came out, I went in alone.

He looked like an elongated garden gnome and was full of nervous energy, making nonstop small talk while I suppressed my discomfort with a smile. Eventually, he calmed down a little and started posing proper 'get to know you' questions. He asked me what I liked doing in my spare time. I said going to the movies.

'You know the 1940s film star Esther Williams?' he asked me.

Sure I did. I was a nerdy girl who liked watching old movies with her mother and sister on the weekends.

'They used to censor the synchronised swimming scenes in her films if any of the movements suggested the opening and closing of a vagina.'

Even at the time, this struck me as a fairly offbeat response to a teenage girl saying, 'I like movies.'

I never went back and neither did Mum, who remained tight-lipped about her session. I wonder now whether she mainly wanted me to go to therapy, and the dual session was in fact, a ruse.

That said, we saw that psychiatrist again and again for years, albeit not willingly.

After my session, we returned home from shopping to find an enormous pile of books on our doorstep (poetry, novels, autobiographies, an eclectic collection) and a note from Dr Gnome saying he hoped I would enjoy reading these and talking about them the next time he saw me.

He would drop by unannounced in the evenings every couple of months and insist on tea and manic conversation with my mother, who didn't know how to get rid of him without making a scene. Until he tried to show her his swollen genitals, made purple by his recent vasectomy. Then she told him not to come around anymore.

He never knocked on the door again, but on occasion he would park outside the house at night. He'd sit there for hours, staring in the general direction of my mother's window. After a few years of this, he disappeared.

Mum never tried to find a new therapist for me. If I ever suggested she might benefit from therapy, she reminded me about Dr Gnome. 'Most psychiatrists also see a psychiatrist,' she would say, as clear evidence that there must be an intractable problem with the profession.

When I was twenty-one I had my first real, productive experience with therapy. It was the early 1990s, and if you think there's a stigma around mental health now, it's peanuts compared to what it was like back then. I'm not sure I told anyone I was in therapy, not even my closest friends.

Faye was a psychiatrist working out of one of the bigger public hospitals. Mum had taken me to see her a couple of times in my early teens, during a short but particularly intense year in which I developed an eating disorder. I tracked Faye down and made an appointment.

I was on a mission to 'fix myself'. Dad was living overseas. I might hear from him once or twice a year, on my birthday and at Christmas – never a phone call but a greeting card with a cheque inside it. I was estranged from Mum and, as a result, couldn't see my sister. Mum and I had been fighting with increasing ferocity since Dad walked out, and there was no other family around. It was just me in a rented room in a house with some university mates, trying hard to stay afloat while I finished my Honours dissertation.

I would never have said it out loud, but I felt like being isolated from my immediate family meant there was something clearly wrong with me. I'd been difficult from the moment I burst out of my mother's womb. Too much energy, too much fight, too many demands. The violence in our house was almost always triggered by me: something I had done, something I had said. I was the reason our family wasn't happy, the reason our home wasn't peaceful.

My sister was a quiet, kind, dutiful daughter, much less likely to trigger anyone. I was defiant. Less likely to take no for an answer. And, once I hit my teens, happy to start yelling back at my mother. Questioning her views about the world, her ideas of right or wrong. Running away.

After a particularly bad fight when I was still in high school, my mother said to me in a tone of grave concern, 'I'm worried about you Rebecca. You are so difficult to be with, I think you might grow up to be very lonely. No real friends or anyone who will be able to live with you.'

I didn't want that. I wanted to be easy. If I was easy, then people would like me. Love me, even.

I was going to therapy to learn how to be easier.

Faye's area of expertise was adolescent psychology, but because I'd seen her as a teenager, she was prepared to see me as an adult. I went regularly to talk, and she listened. She didn't say much, like all good therapists do at the beginning. No manic small talk or comments about pulsating vaginas. After about six sessions, I asked her the question I had been wanting to ask since we first started meeting.

'So, what's wrong with me and how can I fix it? I'm open to taking medication, I just don't want to be on drugs for a long time.'

I can't remember if she smiled at me in a benevolent way – I imagine she might have – but she said something like this.

'There is nothing really wrong with you, Rebecca. You are certainly more reactive than other people because you've grown up in a dysfunctional family. But even if your parents seek help for their issues, you will probably be in and out of therapy for a very long time. Maybe for the rest of your life.'

The thought of a lifelong reliance on psych meds was my greatest concern, but a lifelong reliance on therapy had never occurred to me. I didn't want to believe what she was saying.

However, there was one saving grace.

Faye was the first adult I trusted who said it might not be all my fault.

*

I continued to see Faye for a year or so, until I went overseas on a student exchange. I saw another therapist in my mid-twenties, when I developed a fear of flying. She was into cognitive behavioural therapy and taught me how breathing and different ways of thinking could control my panic attacks during turbulence. Within twelve months I was flying again, albeit with the help of a few Valium. Therapy for me was like spraining an ankle: treatment for a few months and then you're good to go until your next injury.

For years I was 'therapy free'. I thought I was 'cured', and my life was a testament that I was fixed: PhD finished, new job, my first book published. I met a man, fell in love and got married. Flew to Italy for a holiday. Got pregnant quickly and had a baby. Then, in my thirties, a series of curveballs – fertility issues, mainly – sent me back, somewhat reluctantly, to therapy again. A doctor at our local clinic referred me to Karen.

Karen ticked the boxes for me. Her office was in the next suburb. She was a woman. And the GP said she was an expert in perinatal psychiatry. By that stage my eldest daughter was around three and I was desperate to be pregnant again.

From the very beginning, I felt comfortable in her presence. She had a well-trimmed bob, twinkling blue eyes and an open face. She smiled easily. When I look back at our first encounter, I recall thinking, *This person is going to help me sort things out quickly so I can stop coming here and get back to my life.*

She says I told her I needed therapy because I needed a place where I could go to cry. That there was no time in my current schedule to cry.

She remembers too that in the first years of seeing her, when she would start to wrap up the session I would jump up and run out of the room, apologising that I'd taken up too much of her time.

I always thought there was someone who needed her more than I did waiting outside.

For years I would see Karen in fits and starts. I'd go regularly for a few months then stop, then something would happen and I would ask to see her again. She took my lack of commitment to consistent therapy in her stride. Only after a few years did she broach the subject, and only then as a comment to my then husband, who I'd dragged along to a session so he could understand me better.

'I think Rebecca should consider coming to see me more often, because I believe she has been under-treated.'

Under-treated? News to me. I thought I was the poster girl for regular therapy. Between my stints with Faye in my twenties, dealing with my fear of flying and then connecting with Karen, I felt like I was doing more therapy than anyone I knew.

By the time I was headed towards fifty, I was seeing Karen once a month; sometimes more. I would always find things to say, and I would always leave feeling better than I had when I arrived. Working with her, I developed a solid understanding of how much the violence and abuse of my childhood had shaped me as a person. I supported my formal therapy with years of reading books, and articles online, listening to podcasts and talking to friends.

Karen was a godsend, and yet I was becoming frustrated at my lack of progress. I was still angry all the time, still making the same mistakes in relationships, just with different people. Still blowing up. Still pushing myself to the edge in every aspect of my life. I was struggling to rest, incapable of self-compassion. I desperately wanted to know I had finished the work. I'd read all that 'there is no out, only through' palaver in the books about healing. But how long was through? Would it take me to retirement? The nursing home? The grave?

The personal and professional challenges came thick and fast in the last few years of my forties. Each brought a new revelation about myself, and the hope that I was close to some kind of summit of personal growth. But instead, each time, I felt as if I had crawled over the edge of a plateau, fingernails bleeding, panting heavily, only to see the clouds part and reveal another peak waiting to be scaled. I was exhausted. At times I dragged myself to therapy, feeling like I was going through the motions.

There were certain moments, too, when no amount of therapy or reading or walking or working or cleaning or any of the many self-regulating behaviours I had developed over time could make me feel better.

Without any knowledge about how trauma impacts the body, I used to say that it was as if I had been poisoned, as if some kind of malevolent by-product of what happened to me as a child had taken liquid form and was now surging through my bloodstream.

When I returned from the Camino, I started pondering a life without therapy. Why wasn't I getting there faster? Was I wasting my time, and Karen's?

And I started to think, maybe therapy wasn't working for me anymore.

*

When I was ten years old, we moved from our quiet little house near the sea and our ever-present Italian grandparents to Sydney. Dad had been offered the first of many career-making opportunities to work on a report on Aboriginal customary law for the Australian Law Reform Commission. We might as well have been moving to another country, Sydney was so different from Adelaide. It was a big, expensive city, and we knew no-one. We packed all our possessions into a truck, which was driven to Sydney and parked in a warehouse that promptly burnt to the ground.

Whether it was arson or just an accident, the cause was irrelevant, the impact the same. Before we had even left Adelaide, almost everything we had was gone. Dad, his thoughts always buried in his work, had neglected to insure the contents of the van.

The day after we learned about the fire, we went to Target. My father was already in Sydney, working, and so my mother was alone, filling a trolley with everyday household items, knowing she needed to replace what we'd lost with cheap alternatives. We needed everything. I picked up a vegetable peeler and thought about our old one. Burnt plastic now, twisted, never to glide across the surface of a potato again. I put it back with the other pristine peelers and tried not to think about the state of my toys.

I looked back at this move from Adelaide to Sydney as the true start of my father's brilliant career and the beginning of the end of my parents' marriage.

In Sydney, Dad disappeared into his work in a way I'd never seen before. He had always been obsessive, working twelve-hour days, pausing only on a Sunday afternoon to relax. But with this move, his workaholism rose to new levels. The bedtime reading stopped. No more mad kisses or walks to get gelato. He had always been frightening and unpredictable, but his work stress increased so dramatically, the sound of his key turning in the front door would cause my body to stiffen involuntarily, a reflex that would remain with me years after his departure.

In Adelaide my mother had a small group of teacher friends, and her parents helped with domestic tasks, childcare and cooking. In Sydney she was alone, working and looking after us. She was miserable, and I felt it, though she tried hard to make it jolly for us. Sometimes on a Sunday, she would bake a cake and fill a thermos with hot chocolate and we would drive down to Bronte Beach, sit on a rug and eat and drink and look at the ocean. My mother loved the ocean, even though she couldn't swim. She could look at it for hours. I still remember the taste of the cake, the hot drinks and the salt in the sea breeze.

Other weeks she struggled. She spent much more time in her nightgown during the day. She'd lie in the middle of my parents' bed watching a small colour TV with our new cat, Sophie, by her side. Sophie wasn't a moggy like Buffy (who had run away, never to be seen again), but a pedigree. She was a sleek, calm animal and she brought my mother solace in her isolation and her simmering rage at being left in this new city, without financial resources or support, to work, run a house and raise children.

This first stint in Sydney was the first time my parents fought in front of us. It happened a handful of times our first year in that city. Then one afternoon I walked out of my room and saw my mother's luggage packed by the door. She was leaving, apparently. Going back to Adelaide and leaving us to be looked after by Dad. I'm not sure what scared me more, her leaving or us being left alone with Dad, with no-one to intervene during one of his inevitable meltdowns. Perhaps her intention to leave was real, perhaps it was a threat to make him pay attention. They fought about it throughout the night. My sister and I sat in our room straining to hear what they were saying. He placated her. She unpacked her bags.

It was in Sydney that I really started to eat and eat and eat. My father would regularly entertain his colleagues at our home and my mother was expected to cater for large groups of people on her own. She found cooking a bore and a burden, and the legal academics my father was so desperate to cultivate seemed to dismiss her as an uninteresting school teacher.

She put on a decent spread of Italian food for these parties, and would rely on Sara Lee cheesecakes topped with fresh fruit for dessert. My mother fumed over the sink, washing dishes, while my father networked with his peers. Out of my father's view, I would steal slice after slice of cheesecake and scoff them quickly in the bathroom, eating until I was sick and sometimes having to throw it up in the toilet afterwards. In the morning, I would wake up hungry, my father would already be at the office and my mother would be left with the aftermath.

This is when I learned to be really good at cleaning.

After school one day in that first horrible year, after her aborted attempts to flee to Adelaide, my mother pulled me into her room, not in a fit of rage but in quiet determination, triggered by something I can't remember and that she didn't share. Perhaps it was seeing me walk towards her idling car at school pick-up, the biggest girl in my year. There was nothing remotely cute about my expanding flesh by then.

She asked me to strip down to my underpants and led me towards the full-length mirror in front of her bed. She stood next to me and our eyes met in our shared reflection. I had no choice but to look at my chest, where breasts were starting to develop like pinched dumplings. Until that moment I had refused to look at them properly, dressing quickly each morning, still wearing a white cotton singlet rather than a training bra. As a girl who was horrified rather than excited by Judy Blume novels, I was in denial about the onset of puberty. Her face was impassive, her voice businesslike.

'I want you to have a good look at how fat you are, Rebecca.'

I didn't disagree with her, and I don't recall saying anything. She didn't make me stand there for long. Like with my father's physical attacks, it's hard to nail the duration. I put my clothes on as soon as I was given permission to do so, then slunk into my room and thought about what was for dinner.

Every full-length mirror I've seen myself in since has had a kind of faded daguerreotype of my pudgy, almost-naked body in the background, like those ghost photos from the nineteenth century.

Clearly, if I was thinner, my mother would be happier.

A slice of Christmas cake in the sun

In 2022 I had my first Christmas alone and it was less awful than I'd feared. With no Dad or Mum, and my sister with her husband's clan, I suggested to my ex that the children spend Christmas with his family, who celebrated the occasion with all the trimmings. He agreed, and picked them up from my place on Christmas Eve.

I woke up on Christmas Day and walked the dog, then came home and made myself peanut butter toast (I'd read somewhere that it can make you feel happy). Pottered around. Had a bath. Packed some leftovers in my backpack and drove to the edge of the CBD. I was planning to walk into the city, down towards the Opera House and back, about a three-hour tramp. It was perfect weather, hot but not humid with a cool breeze. There were more people walking around than I expected. I sat on a bench in Hyde Park and ate some leftover Christmas cake from a party I'd thrown a few days before, then drove home and lay on the couch reading, the dog by my side, until bedtime.

Legendary British food writer Elizabeth David once wrote that if she had her way, Christmas Day 'would consist of an omelette and cold ham and a nice bottle of wine at lunchtime, and a smoked salmon sandwich with a glass of champagne'.[5] Women of her generation rarely got their way. Women of my mother's generation didn't either. And even for me, Christmas was never a consistently magical time.

Before having children, I dreamed of creating joyous Christmas events for my family. I collected Christmas ornaments before I even had a tree to decorate. When the kids arrived, I would plan for months in advance, working out the Christmas catering and gifts and decorations. I sent cards. But after a decade, it became harder to put in this effort. After hosting Christmas lunches, I would suggest my ex take the kids for a drive while I cleaned up all the mess. It would take hours. I'd think of my mother fuming in the kitchen while my father swanned around chatting to people at the many parties he insisted they host. My heart went out to her as I scrubbed roasting trays, exhausted.

Once Mum was in her sixties and free of hosting obligations, she sometimes tried to opt out of the holiday altogether. I turned myself inside out trying to make Christmas a feel-good family moment. I prepared the food my mother loved – the cakes and puddings from the island of Elba where her parents were born, her favourite Baci chocolate, chocolate-covered nuts and lots of French champagne. I agonised over what gifts to get her. But there was always a real chance she wouldn't front. I would call her a few days before to confirm she was coming, only to have her not turn up because she was 'feeling unwell'. Or she would stay for a short time and then leave without saying goodbye when I was in another room. Stupidly, I never asked her about the cause of this confusing behaviour. I just thought I needed to try harder.

A slice of Christmas cake in the park on a bench in the sun didn't seem so bad in comparison.

In the week that followed that first-time-alone Christmas Day, I had a lot of free time on my hands.

It was tempting to cram a big project into this empty time – another book, a spring clean, a new skill like making ravioli. The kind of all-encompassing project people like me take on so they don't accidentally find themselves relaxing. I woke up the day after Boxing Day and messaged a few friends who I knew might be around and at a loose end. Almost immediately, one got back to me suggesting lunch. We met at an unremarkable pub, one of the only ones open on Oxford Street during that eerily quiet time between Christmas and New Year's Eve.

I'd known Abby for over twenty years. We met through her husband, who was a classmate from university days. From the moment she walked into my apartment for our first coffee date we clicked. We always had a lot to talk about, with overlapping interests and a similar world view. She had a soothing energy and a keen sense of humour. Abby came from a high-powered family of inherited money. Over the years, the occasional comment or dark joke made me wonder if we shared the same kind of damage, but I never probed.

We sat across from each other in the Paddington pub booth. She ordered a glass of champagne for us both and we picked at some food.

After some small talk, she asked me, 'How are you?'

There was something about her tone, the genuine concern in her voice, and her gaze, which fell across me like a light blanket.

I resisted the urge to downplay everything that had happened during the year and simply said, 'I've decided not to see my mother anymore.'

'Oh my god,' she said, 'you're allowed to do that? How amazing!'

*

Over lunch, I gave Abby the whistlestop tour of my family history and what had led to my decision to sever all contact with my mother.

She listened and nodded. She thankfully didn't engage in the usual 'but she's your mother', 'you need to forgive her for you' or even worse, 'life's too short' platitudes that I feared would follow my confession. As a daughter, deciding to cut your mother out of your life seems like an unthinkable act of betrayal, almost anti-feminist.

Abby responded not with pop psychology about forgiveness and the importance of family, but with stories of her own.

And then she told me about Julia and her experience with MDMA.

She'd met Julia through a friend at a party. Julia was a healer with decades of experience using plant-based medicines, whose practice over the last few years had been centred around MDMA. Abby had travelled to see Julia in her home in the

Northern Rivers region of New South Wales for a session, which took all day and was clearly revelatory.

The story intrigued me. Abby wasn't a drug taker in any recreational sense. She was sensible and grounded and evidence based in everything she did. So, the fact that she'd had this profound experience on MDMA with an underground practitioner made me take it seriously.

In the books that Nicky had encouraged me to read, and in other books I'd picked up since then, like Gabor Maté's *The Myth of Normal*, the use of drugs like MDMA and psilocybin is discussed at length as having great potential in addressing unresolved trauma.

Abby was convinced I would find Julia and MDMA useful. She offered to introduce me via the closed messaging app Signal.

MDMA was an illegal drug, and what Julia was doing was also illegal. And yet, none of that deterred me. I thought it was worth exploring.

*

A few days later, I found myself exchanging emails with Julia on the secure email server Proton. Before she agreed to meet for a chat online, she gave me a lot of background information about the process and sent me a lengthy questionnaire to fill out.

I didn't clock it at the time, but I realise now that she was trying to work out if I was the right fit for the therapy. Was I ready?

She sent me numerous pages explaining how the process worked. Namely, that the drug floods the amygdala with a wave of serotonin. This subdues your fight or flight response, allowing you to explore your past experiences without the usual reactivity.

Julia's papers emphasised the process rather than the drug, because she wasn't selling me MDMA like a dealer in a nightclub, she was involving me in a process with an important lead-up, and an even more important integration process afterwards.

In the weeks before the first session she and I spoke a few times to explore what I wanted to achieve. There were other kinds of prep work too. I would need to load up on vitamin C and magnesium. No recreational drug taking or alcohol for a few weeks prior. In the two days before the session I should take an amino acid called L-tryptophan that converts to serotonin, to offset the dip that occurs a few days after (those 'eccy Tuesday' feels I remember friends speaking about in my twenties).

A light breakfast on the day, no caffeine or other stimulants. The session would run from 10 am to 4 pm or possibly longer – an extraordinarily long period to be high with a stranger, or so I thought.

I would take one capsule of the drug at the start, and then she would offer me a second dose after a few hours.

Then, in the week after, more L-Tryptophan, B and C vitamins and magnesium. Melatonin or a sleep aid if needed. And lots of self-care. Good food, gentle exercise, time in nature, creative pursuits, and so on.

'Perhaps do not schedule anything demanding soon afterwards, and surround yourself with gentle company,' Julia's notes suggested.

Like a good girl, I went to the vitamin shop, booked a massage and took a few days leave from work.

As I read back through Julia's information, what strikes me is that she didn't over promise. The drug was a facilitator of a process that would not 'cure' me. What I brought into it, the work I was prepared to do before and after, that's what mattered.

The questionnaire she asked me to fill out was remarkably detailed, more than you might complete for a medical professional. Several pages outlining my mental and physical health information, family history, current employment and living arrangements. If I was taking any medication for anything.

After that, I was to write a 'Letter to Self', which would help me articulate what I wanted from the process. I could share it with her or not. Why was I choosing to do this work now? What were the outcomes I wanted to see with the support of this work? What would the change I was looking for look like? Feel like?

That 'Letter to Self' sits on my desktop. I read it from time to time. In it, I was remarkably open about how I wasn't coping, how I was stuck. I would have told even my dearest friends that while my life was challenging, I was happy, fulfilled and exactly where I needed to be. But in response to a series of direct questions, that front of self-assurance fell away. I wrote:

> *When I am not distracted by work or friends I am churning over the events of my childhood and how the relationship with my mother and other important people in my life deteriorated to this point. How I contributed. How unaddressed trauma contributed. Emotions are more like anger and resentment than sadness or regret.*
>
> *'I'd like to be able to think about my past and present in ways where I don't relive and continue to embed those negative feelings. I'd like to be able to reflect on what's happened in a way that feels more compassionate to all involved, including myself. Rather than just punishing and hyper critical. I get flashes of that in my thinking but never in a sustained way.*

I wrote that I was committed to a new approach to healing, but that I was finding it hard, and time-consuming, and lonely.

That I was looking for insight and compassion in equal measure.

I must have said all the right things, because she agreed to a first meeting. We had a Zoom chat one afternoon, me in my study at home and her in her sunroom. I don't remember much about that first discussion. She had a calming voice, shoulder-length light hair, beautiful blue eyes, and the screen was lit up by the sun shining through the sliding doors of her country home. She apologised for being late, she had to hang the laundry out to dry before evening.

We talked through the process in detail, reiterating that she would offer me a second dose of the MDMA after a few hours.

'It's up to you if you want the second dose or not,' she told me.

'Has anyone ever refused?' I asked out of interest.

'Rarely,' she told me.

Clearly this shit was good.

'I don't work with people in the midst of crisis,' she told me. The process was far more efficacious when the immediate crisis had passed and when the nervous system was not in 'arrest mode', she explained. The fact that I was in secure employment, secure accommodation, accessing consistent therapy, surrounded by friends, in good health and that the death, divorce and disruption of the last few years were in the rear-view mirror all made me a good candidate.

We ended the meeting by confirming a time and a place for session one.

She would be visiting Sydney in a few weeks, and would come to me.

Session one

The days before my first MDMA session, the kids were with their dad and I was lost in work – focus groups and report writing. I had to travel interstate for meetings with clients. I returned home the night before feeling tired but relaxed.

As I settled into bed with a novel, I wondered whether instead of reading, I should learn more about the physical side effects of MDMA. I was curiously uncurious about what would happen, given I had never taken the drug before. I had surrendered myself to a process that I trusted, even though it was somewhat mysterious to me. I googled side effects anyway, just to make it easier to drift off to sleep. Muscle tightness, decreased appetite, nausea, sweating and feeling cold. I had the muscle tightness and sweating anyway, thanks to perimenopause. The rest sounded like a mild case of the flu.

I returned to my book, but only got five pages into *Les Misérables*, putting it down at the part where Fantine leaves Cosette in the custody of the cruel Mr and Mrs Thénardier.

The morning of the session could not have been more beautiful – clear skies, warm but not too warm. I walked the dog to the kennels; he was a barking, licking cavoodle whose energy I suspected would not be a welcome addition to the MDMA experience. On the walk back home, I started wondering, not about the seemingly manageable physical side effects, but about the behaviour the MDMA might unleash. Would I completely lose control?

My point of reference was not personal experience but observation at clubs when I was in my twenties. I saw MDMA as a drug for people looking to party. One that prompted extroverted behaviour, not introspective thought. Would I be gyrating on the living room ottoman during the session? *'Doof, doof, doof … and there was that one time my dad threw me into an open closet … doof, doof, doof … everybody dance now …'*

Julia had instructed me to fast, so I skipped breakfast and even my compulsive three cups of coffee before 9 am and waited. At this point, my main anxiety was about the food I had organised for my guest. I had been fretting about it for days.

How do you cater for such an occasion? Martha Stewart remains frustratingly silent on this issue. Sushi? Charcuterie board? Or something more substantial, like lasagne?

Since our first online discussion, Julia and I had messaged each other a few times, and we'd had one more pre-session chat. She'd asked if I had any final questions before we met, and the only one that sprang to mind was, 'What food should I make for you? If you are with me all day, I'll need to cater. What should I prepare?'

'Oh, you won't want to eat. I'll bring something for myself.'

'No, please let me organise something for you.'

I had settled on a roast chicken and a few salads, iced tea, cakes, and a plate of salted caramels I'd bought at a local chocolate shop.

I wondered whether my over-catering tendencies could be attributed to being a proud Italian or a chronic people pleaser.

The doorbell rang and I opened the door to a slender woman with sandals and a backpack.

There is always a momentary jolt of adjustment when you meet someone in person who you are familiar with from Zoom meetings. It's hard to get the complete vibe of someone online. Julia's vibe was soporific in a way that would usually annoy me.

It's not that I hate hippies. It's just their earthiness and yoga-teacher voices provoke an immediate and over-the-top irritation in me. Their softness brings out my hard edges. It is as if they aren't ashamed of their vulnerability.

So I looked at Julia, at her make-up-free face and her ankle bracelets and her calm voice and flowing movements and for a split second I thought, *What the fuck am I doing with this person?*

Her vibe was hippie but her backpack meant business. Sturdy, black, it looked like it was made from Kevlar. After a tour of the house and the food I'd prepared, we sat in my lounge room and I watched her unpack.

A laptop and speaker to play her carefully curated soundtrack for the many hours we would be together. A candle. A notepad and pen so she could write down whatever I said under the influence. A zip-lock bag with the 'medicine'. And scales – not the kind you use for baking but scales I had never seen before, something a compounding chemist might use.

Where was I most comfortable, she asked me. Easy. The long grey couch I had bought a few months ago. It was large enough to stretch out flat, legs straight, shavasana style. Sturdy enough for regular use, but the brushed cotton and big pillows made it a place where you could fall asleep, even if dogs and children were sharing the space.

She pulled an armchair up close to the couch and asked for a blanket.

'Are you cold?' I asked. 'Do you want me to put on the heater?'

'Not for me,' she said with a smile I was now familiar with. 'For you. You might get cold.' I remembered the symptom list from the night before.

I sat on the couch while she measured the two doses using the serious scales and put the tiny, white MDMA crystals into capsules. Apparently, the taste is acrid if consumed directly. More crystals for the first burst, less for the second, just like she had explained.

She started the music – rhythmic, world music beats like you get in a boho spa – then lit the candle. The burnt wood of the flame's aftermath filled the air. She sat cross-legged in the armchair, cupped the capsules in her hand and closed her eyes.

'We give thanks to the sassafras tree, whose roots provide us with this medicine and the gift of love, compassion and insight into our lives, that helps us heal and walk away from what no longer serves us.'

As she recited the blessing, cynicism flickered inside me for a split second, the same internal eye roll that stops me from saying 'namaste' at the end of a yoga class. And yet, the blessing made me feel like what was about to happen was fundamentally unlike the kind of recreational drug-taking I had been used to.

I swallowed the first capsule and laid back against the couch pillows, my legs outstretched. I was facing away from the TV mounted on the wall, staring towards the front door. Through the glass pane between the door and the wall I could see cobwebs, previously unnoticed by me, in the corner where the door meets the roof.

It took a great deal of restraint not to jump up, grab a feather duster and sweep them away.

I took a deep breath. It was a rare thing for me to lie down during the day, and the fact there was a guest in my home and I was facing away from the television was unsettling. I kept looking at the cobwebs. I took another breath.

I worried Julia would be bored. The social researcher in me switched on. I wanted to know about her life. How had she arrived at this kind of work? What is her clientele like? More women than men? Young, old, rich, not so rich? What kinds of agonies has she seen unfurl before her on couches across the country and around the world?

I took another breath.

She was definitely bored.

The first track ended and a similar one started up, more rhythmic drumming but with voices this time.

I closed my eyes. Maybe the drug won't work on me. Maybe I'll just have a forced nap. That would be nice enough. I felt tired.

I broke the silence but didn't open my eyes.

'I'm not sure I have anything to say at the moment. I'm worried you might be bored.'

Julia reminded me she wasn't necessarily there to ask me questions like my therapist. She was there to guide and respond to whatever emerged. Apparently, some people are silent throughout the whole session, lying still as tears stream from their eyes. Others start talking and don't stop.

I can't recall whether it was during the third song or the fourth when it happened. Julia's notes say I took the drug at 10.46 and by 11.01 I said I was 'feeling it'.

It started like the familiar feeling from a joint or a strong painkiller, that comforting tug towards the ground, away from pain and tension. And then it quickly became something else.

Have you ever laid down on the beach where the waves crawl across the sand, and let them slowly drag you into the ocean until you are no longer on the shore but floating on the surface?

It was like that, only instead of floating on cold water, I was held by a warm body of emotion and memory. And then I submerged, and was slowly dragged by a rip-tide that should have frightened me but didn't. A rip-tide that moved me from memory to memory to memory in unexpected ways.

At first, this rip-tide dragged me into a memory I've recalled a few times a week since my daughter Stella was born.

But the MDMA made me remember – made me *feel* – this memory differently from the way I usually do.

Stella is a twin, the first one out of the womb and the only child the hospital staff gave me to hold after I had my C-section. Her sister Sadie wasn't breathing and so she went straight from my body into an incubator and then into an ambulance, sent to the only available NICU ward on the other side of town.

I was full to the brim with the drugs from the epidural when they put Stella on my chest to hold. It was a moment I usually describe as pure happiness. I'd thrashed my way through blood, pain, needles and piles of money to get to that moment. This was the first memory that the MDMA rip-tide pulled me towards, but the feeling I experienced through the drug was not pure happiness, but something else.

The absence of terror.

I had, in fact, been terrified every second of that long, hard pregnancy. Terrified that the babies would die. That my tired, overwhelmed, unloved body would kill them. I had successfully suppressed those feelings, not just while I was pregnant with the twins but ever since.

The MDMA made me understand that, made me feel that moment differently.

I sat in the memory refashioned by the drug. Eyes closed, all awareness of my surroundings had melted away. I couldn't feel the couch underneath me or the temperature of the air around me. I only barely registered the soundscape of Julia's music, when one song shifted into the next.

What I could feel was the light weight of my daughter on the left side of my chest, above the heart. I sat in that memory for seconds, minutes, maybe more. It was impossible to judge at the time.

Then, gently, the rip-tide pulled me away, towards something that could not be described as a memory at all, unless you believe babies have memories that can be stored and recalled.

I walked into a sparse, dark room with one window and a crib in the centre. It was as if I had gotten up from the bed with Stella and walked into this second scene alone. The crib was wooden, empty except for a mattress and a baby. The baby was me. I was neither happy nor sad. Just still, silent. My mother was standing in the corner of the room, looking like I've seen her in family photos as a young woman, slender with long dark brown hair parted in the middle, wearing a 1970s-style dress. She was staring at the baby, not with love nor malice but impassivity. Still, silent, like the baby. I walked over to the crib, picked myself up and left the room. I lay down again on the hospital bed, restored Stella to her original place on my left side and put the baby, me as I was in 1972, on the right side.

The drug wasn't yet strong enough to stop me from an inner snort at the cliché. Embracing my inner child. Trying to make up for the traumas of my childhood through my own actions as a mother.

This drug was good. I would never have let myself conjure up something this banal.

Looking back at this moment, it's the impassive face of my mother that I return to. How familiar the expression was. The same 'dead' face I would see over my father's shoulder as he raged at me, when he would grab me by the shoulders and shake me or hit me or throw me. The same face when I came to her for help at any crisis point in my life.

You need help. Part of me wants to help you. But I'm not going to help you.

Lying on the hospital bed with the two babies, I wondered, *What next? Where should I go now?* Some part of my brain was still trying to control what was happening, trying to get through a psychological 'to-do list', the way I plough through tasks at the shopping centre. But as Julia had told me, the process has a wisdom of its own. I could no more guide it consciously than I could force a broken-down trolley through the supermarket aisles.

I was still trying to second-guess where the drug might pull me when I found myself floating over a blistering hot desert scene, red earth and a cloudless blue sky, quintessentially outback Australia, a place I'd never visited and had only seen in pictures. A voice I didn't recognise, a man's voice, reassuring and low, told me to 'let go'. And I did, surrendering. I sank deeper.

In that deeper state I could both visualise and feel something open up inside me. A slowly churning, greyish whirlpool. It was as if it was made of millions of flecks of sand. I peered into it; it was bottomless. I know it sounds contradictory that I could look into it while it was inside me, but it was possible. I knew, I felt, that the whirlpool was an endless pit of sadness lying just beneath the anger I had been feeling so acutely. This was the whirligig of my Camino hike, revealed in its true form. Not anger, but a deep sorrow.

The whirlpool was not sadness for myself, what I'd gone through, but for my mother. My father too. A limitless well of sorrow and compassion for what they'd experienced in their own lives.

I believe they were never really taught how to love. How lamentable that was. For them. For us as a family.

I stared into the whirlpool for what felt like ages.

Suddenly I was aware that my neck felt wet. Perhaps I was cold, but also sweating, like you do when you have a temperature. I touched my face with one hand and realised it was wet with tears. It wasn't the kind of crying I was used to, hot tears of frustration and angry sobs, but a steady stream of noiseless tears.

I returned my wet hand to my side and found myself in the midst of another memory. Not so much a suppressed memory, but a memory I had forgotten to remember. I was six years old. We had returned to Oxford, England, for one of the many sabbaticals my father would take us on, to the town of my birth and the place where he was determined one day to hold the prestigious chair in international law. I was sick with a very bad flu. I was lying in a single bed in the room I shared with my sister in our rented accommodation, hovering in that half-conscious, half-delirious state of high fever. It was evening, or the middle of the night – that, I am fuzzy on. What I can recall with clarity is my mother sitting by the bed, close to me, holding a damp, cool flannel to my forehead. In the dim glow of the bedside lamp, I could see her face in the half-light. The Roman nose, high cheekbones and forehead, thin lips and dark eyes. My eyes were closed, but I would open them every now and then to look at her. To check she was still there, close to me.

I remember the look on her face. One of concentrated, undistracted concern. While I felt awful because of the fever, I felt something else, something that only under the MDMA thrall could I properly identify.

I felt safe.

I didn't want the fever to end.

I sat in the memory of my mother's soft attention and the cool cloth on my head.

'This is what love feels like,' I said to Julia.

Did I want more of the medicine, Julia asked.

'Yes please. Could I have a blanket too?'

The water felt cold and strange as I swallowed capsule number two.

I lay back, breathing steadily, eyes closed.

'This stuff is magic,' I said to Julia.

I turned over on my side, my face still wet, my hands folded underneath my cheek.

'My sister. My sister. My sister,' I said.

*

I am the eldest of my father's seven children. He had four wives, one after another with barely a pause for breath in between them. The age gap between his first and his last child is forty-three years.

The gap between myself and my sister, Emily, is only three years. We grew up together, apart. No-one else in the world understands what we went through. But for most of our lives it was almost impossible for us to talk honestly about anything that really mattered.

Emily was born an angelically beautiful and placid child. Her birth was easy. She was born in Adelaide, where Mum was happiest in the warmth of the South Australian sun and with the support of her parents. Nonna was there to help raise my sister, and to help my mother in whatever way she could.

Emily had none of the vim I had as a toddler. Where I was energetic to the point of being bumptious, Emily was placid, almost lethargic. Mum would say as a baby I would grip on to her so tightly she could hold her arms up in the air and I wouldn't fall. In contrast, she had to hold my sister with both arms and all her strength, and still she would often slide off her hip and down her leg.

So my sister and I were antithetical from the beginning. Her hair was straight, mine was curly. She was thin, I wasn't. She avoided conflict, I was prepared to argue the toss. She liked green olives and I liked black olives. Well, maybe not. Maybe over time we just decided to be as different as possible because, like I said, we were growing up together, apart.

It always felt to me like my sister was born kind. Mum used to say that if she gave Emily a snack like a sweet biscuit, she would take it and hold out her other hand and say, 'Becca.' That my name was her first word. That might not be true, but it feels true. Those stories were usually the precursor to Mum telling me that I had been a bad sister from the beginning.

'You were always so horrible to her. All she wanted you to do was to protect her.'

Mum wasn't entirely wrong. I was horrible to Emily, more so than the usual older-sister meanness. I resented her. Her arrival meant the already scant amount of attention and love I was receiving had been halved. She was everything I felt my parents wanted me to be. I'd tell her she was adopted. I'd lock her out of the house. I'd hit her. Slap her. Ignore her. Boss her around. Ridicule her interests and hobbies.

It's funny how siblings in families like mine can turn on each other, when logic suggests they'd fare better banding together. And yet even a shallow dive into the literature on sibling rivalry in unhappy families makes me realise that Katniss and Prim are the exception rather than the rule. Still, I beat myself up for years – and still do – that I couldn't be Katniss. As a kid, I'd have let Emily walk into the Hunger Games alone.

In my lifelong focus on my parents, I forget how important my sister has been in my life. It should have come as no surprise that she would play a starring role in my first MDMA trip, and yet I was surprised. There was so much other shit to work through.

*

'My sister. My sister. My sister.'

I said the words out loud to Julia even before the memory kicked in. Another recollection, not repressed so much as forgotten.

Emily and I attended the same primary school when we first moved to Sydney in the early 1980s. By then I was nine going on ten. I felt truly ugly and was full of self-loathing. She was adorable and largely unaware of it. I didn't want her anywhere near me in the playground. I'd ignore her even when we walked in and out of the yard at the beginning and end of the school day.

It was an oppressively hot summer lunchtime in December. Kids ran to and from the bubblers to drink and spray each other. I was loitering around the water trough with my friends when my sister approached me. A rare transgression, given she knew she would be met with indifference at best, hostility at worst.

There is no forgetting her face. Her large brown eyes framed by a bowl haircut she was managing to pull off. She was flushed red.

'Rebecca, I feel really sick.'

'Just get a drink of water,' I said over my shoulder as I walked away.

Later that day, when our mother picked us up, Emily was still flushed, but silent. We drove home and she made her way up to her room on the first floor. After devouring snacks in the kitchen, I went upstairs. She was lying straight and motionless on her bed, staring at the ceiling.

I said something, I can't remember what.

Silence.

I said it louder.

Silence still. She just lay there staring.

She was ignoring me. It was some kind of game, the silent treatment. Screw that. That was my schtick.

I said something horrible to her. No response. I said more terrible stuff. Again, nothing. I went over to her, intending to shove her to get some kind of reaction.

She had a blank expression, was glassy eyed. I realised something was wrong.

I shook her shoulders, not with resentment but growing concern.

'Emily, say something.'

She sat up suddenly and projectile vomited across her bed, splattering me in the process. And then she started to fit. Her head thrown back, her whole body started to shake.

I must have screamed because very quickly Mum came and bustled us into the car and raced us to the doctor. We were an alarming threesome: Emily and I covered in vomit-stained school uniforms and Mum in her nightie and bathrobe. By the time we got to the doctor Emily was conscious, but in shock.

After a short examination, the doctor told us she'd had a febrile convulsion, caused by prolonged fever.

As we drove home, I felt an immense sense of shame. I'd dismissed Emily in the playground, failed to grasp her illness in the car and abused her as she lay unconscious on the bed.

Why had the MDMA led me to this moment? It was spotlighting something I already felt, that I'd been a bad sister and that Emily, a quiet, good, beautiful soul, had suffered as much as I had in that family.

I sat up a little and wiped my eyes.

'I think we might take a break now,' Julia said. 'I might eat something quickly.'

Morning tea? It had only been an hour or so. Clearly this chick was one of those skinny hungry types.

'What time is it?' I asked.

'It's a little past two o'clock.'

Jesus. Three hours had passed and it felt like an hour. Julia had spent most of the past two hours kneeling on the floor with her hand on my back as the rip-tide pulled me here and there.

While she grabbed some food, I went to the toilet and drank some more water, and then for the rest of the session I talked and talked and talked. Julia scribbled notes while I spoke about it all – my sister, my mother, my father, the violence, the cruelty, the moments of joy and closeness, the terrible loneliness, the sense of responsibility I felt for it all. Story after story.

As evening approached, Julia started to wind up the session. I rinsed my face. My friend Michael was coming over to keep me company before bedtime. I wrapped up all the salted caramels and gave them to Julia to take home with her.

As the drug started to wear off, I felt sheepish, like I had burdened her with too much, too quickly. It's like I dumped $8000 worth of trauma on her for a session that had cost me $800.[6]

'I'm sorry,' I said as we were saying our goodbyes. 'That was a lot. Too much maybe.'

'Not at all,' she said with her reassuring smile.

She handed over her handwritten notes and encouraged me to read them later.

'There was a lot that came up, but what stood out for me was that moment you remembered with your mother, where she was caring for you when you were sick. You took that feeling and you elevated that. It's how you can be a mother to your own children.'

Julia shouldered her Kevlar backpack and walked off into the dusk.

I woke up the next day to find out that Australia was the first place in the world to make MDMA therapy legal.

A drug called therapy

MDMA was a mistake.

A mistake, in that it was an accidental by-product created by chemists searching for something other than a drug for people dealing with complex trauma.

In 1912 the German pharmaceutical company Merck was looking for medicines to control bleeding. In the pursuit of that goal, they discovered methylenedioxymethamphetamine. They patented it in 1914, but it sat on a shelf until the mid-1970s.

Except for the CIA's brief flirtation with it as a potential mind control drug during the Cold War.

In 1976, American biochemist Alexander Shulgin was introduced to MDMA by a student he was advising at San Francisco State University. He took it and realised he'd 'discovered' a powerful empathogen, a drug that produces feelings of empathy and connectedness. He went on to develop a new method of making the drug, and then introduced it to his friend Leo Zeff, a psychologist working in Oakland, California.

Zeff started to use small doses as an aid in talk therapy for his clients. Its use grew from there, with an enthusiastic group of psychotherapists using the drug (which was a legal substance at that stage) between 1977 and 1985.[7] Interested scientists started the first important research into how it worked and how it could be used as a therapeutic tool.

MDMA's original name was, in fact, 'therapy'.[8]

MDMA quickly spread from the therapist's office to the nightclub and soon became a hugely popular party drug in cities such as Texas and New York. Its name changed from 'therapy' to 'ecstasy'. And then it spread to the party scene throughout the world.

Political and public attention in the United States, including a particularly influential episode of the talk show *Donahue*, led to scrutiny from law enforcement. In 1985, the Drug Enforcement Administration declared an emergency ban on MDMA, placing it on the list of Schedule I drugs, defined as substances with no currently accepted medical use and a high potential for abuse. Other countries around the world followed suit.

After a long and focused campaign to reverse this decision, spearheaded by organisations like the US nonprofit Multidisciplinary Association for Psychedelic Studies (MAPS), MDMA is now on the verge of becoming a legal and legitimate treatment for chronic mental health problems. There are legal psychedelic clinics in Jamaica and Costa Rica. It's been used to treat patients with severe conditions in Switzerland, Canada and Israel. Clinical trials are being conducted in numerous jurisdictions around the world, including in certain states in the US.[9]

But Australia is the first jurisdiction to make it available to the public. To the surprise of many in my country and around the world, on 3 February 2023, the Australian Therapeutic Goods Association (TGA) published its decision to authorise the use of MDMA for post-traumatic stress disorder that has not responded to treatment. Psychiatrists can prescribe the drug and another drug, the mushroom-derived psilocybin, to their patients.

At the time of writing, this decision remains controversial. There have been allegations that the TGA was lobbied hard, to the point of harassment, by the organisation Mind Medicine.[10] Even those hopeful and open to the therapeutic use of MDMA wonder if we have the resources, skills and understanding of the drug needed to maximise its benefits. There are people – like Julia – who have decades of experience in the context of underground therapy, but that counts for little when it comes to legal clinical practice and government policy. Many of these seasoned, underground practitioners aren't medical doctors; they don't have the authority to prescribe. They wonder if the medical profession is, on the whole, sufficiently educated about trauma or these drugs to be the gatekeepers of its use.

Like I said, I grew up in the 1990s, when the club scene was swimming in 'e'. I remember at the one and only Sydney Gay and Lesbian Mardi Gras I attended, 'e' was everywhere. It makes sense to me now why it has been so popular in a community looking for ceremonies to express love, grief and loss.[11]

But even when I was a clubbing twenty-something, I avoided taking it. To be honest, I was scared off by the ecstasy-related death of a teenager, Anna Wood. The fifteen-year-old took an ecstasy tablet at a rave in Sydney, at a club I'd been to a few times. The next day she died from a cerebral oedema caused by water intoxication. That's when excessive fluid consumption dilutes sodium levels in the blood, causing brain damage. Basically, Anna had consumed too much water, something people dancing away on 'e' for hours can do. Her death was caused by behaviour encouraged by MDMA, rather than by the drug itself. Anna's death was on the front cover of all the newspapers in Australia, held up as an example of how deadly ecstasy could be. I didn't need any further convincing – I steered clear. Little did I know that, despite all the studies and reports about the neurotoxicity of MDMA, it is one of the least harmful drugs out there; far less deadly than alcohol.[12]

In all the media coverage, both positive and negative, about the TGA's decision to authorise the use of MDMA for PTSD, it's the drug itself that gets the attention. What all the coverage ignores is that the drug is simply the key to unlocking something far more important: the process. The lead-up to taking the drug and, more importantly, what comes after.

*

The materials Julia first sent me put a lot of emphasis on the post-trip integration. Not only did she suggest taking time off work and taking vitamins, she also encouraged a number of integration sessions to help work through what the MDMA had surfaced. She wrote: *After our session, it is possible that the experience will have a destabilising effect on you as your system adjusts. You may feel worse before you feel better. As insights unveil themselves you may feel uncomfortable but this is an important and unavoidable process as we move towards a more integrated self. We need to collect that which we neglected, stifled, ignored. Having this context and self-compassion is useful in the weeks after.*

I woke up the next morning to more than just the news of MDMA's endorsement as a drug to treat complex trauma.

I woke up to a surprising stillness.

Not outside my window. I could hear the usual sounds of distant dogs barking, birds, delivery trucks, and traffic.

But inside my head, the whirligig was gone.

Suddenly, I understood how someone could become addicted to a drug.

The churning sadness disguised as anger was gone, but the day was still hard.

I was on leave from work. The children were still with their father. I had very little on my to-do list. Abby was coming to see me for a mid-morning coffee. I had to pick up the dog. I wanted to squeeze in a swim.

As I washed my face and brushed my teeth, I was amazed at how undistracted and unpressured I felt. It was as if I had woken up in another kind of body. The sensations of the cold water, the friction of the brush in my mouth, felt sharper, even though I assumed the drug was largely out of my system. As I walked along my neighbourhood streets to pick up the dog, I noticed how unhurried the pace of my walking was. I am a fast walker. If I am not careful, I find myself walking fifteen steps ahead of my children when we are shopping, turning around and then panicking if I've lost sight of them. But that morning I found myself taking steady steps towards the kennels without even having to remind myself I had no reason to rush and nothing urgent to do.

I came home with the dog and made my way into the kitchen to prepare some breakfast, even though my hunger hadn't fully returned. Before I could get to the fridge to pull out some yoghurt, I was stopped in my tracks by an overwhelming sensation. So overwhelming I had to steady myself with both hands on the cold grey stone benchtop. The sensation was like a wall of water, thick and heavy, like you see in those epic surfing movies with the thrill-seeking, big-wave board riders.

I closed my eyes. I pushed my hands down harder onto the benchtop surface. I locked my knees, reinforced my legs the way you are advised not to when you lift a heavy object. The wall of water was there at my back, heavier by the second. At that moment I had two revelations about this unrelenting pressure bearing down on me.

One: That I had to hold. Lying down and letting it wash over me was not an option. I knew I could do it, that I was strong enough to make my body an immovable barrier between this pressure and whatever was in front of me.

But the weight of it. It was immense. And I felt it. Knew it. Knew it would take its toll on me, and that it already had.

Two: I understood what the wall of water was. A legacy of the pain, violence, isolation and sadness experienced by my parents, their parents, every unknown ancestor along the branches of my family tree who didn't have the capacity, the desire, the opportunity or the tools to recover from what hurt them.

And what lay between that wall and the space in front of me? Not the fridge with the yoghurt I had been planning to eat, but my children. My body was the barrier between that powerful wave and my girls.

My daughters might be splashed from time to time by whatever managed to find a path over my shoulders, but I would hold so they would never feel its full force. I would hold until they were safe.

Finally, I managed to unlock my knees and step forward. The sensation subsided and I stumbled to a kitchen stool to catch my breath.

*

Over the following days the anger returned in increments. I woke up a few days later and the whirligig was back.

Hi honey, I'm home.

I never expected the whirligig not to return, but I felt it differently. Now I knew what it was like not to feel it, and as a result I felt more confident managing it. When it was at its loudest, it was easier to step back and look at it with curiosity rather than get swept up in it.

I had more sessions with Julia over Signal. Long talks with Abby and conversations with friends. I called my therapist's office later that week to request an emergency appointment. I had been avoiding Karen to some extent – I'd cancelled four sessions in a row. Once I'd decided to try the MDMA therapy I didn't want to see her, didn't want to tell her in case she talked me out of it. In case she felt I was cheating on her with another 'process'. Karen managed to squeeze me in over the phone quickly and I spent about forty-five minutes cry-talking to her down the line. My fears about her reaction to my 'affair' with another therapeutic approach were unfounded. She was accepting and interested in my experience.

I spent my evenings on the couch researching complex childhood trauma. The algorithms in my social media picked this up quickly, and soon, instead of the usual promotions for kitchen and cleaning gadgets, videos about trauma started popping up in my feeds. In one of these videos, a therapist delivers a TEDx-style talk about being 'a transitional character' – a person who decides to thwart the contagious effects of trauma in a family. Someone who grows up in an abusive and emotionally destructive environment and finds ways to stop passing that on to their children. This was what I was trying to do, and the speaker in the video told me there was no more important, or more difficult, role to play in life.

Listening to him speak, I was back between the sink and the island, channelling all my strength to create a barrier between the wave and the girls. Acknowledging the strain and loneliness of it, but aware that yielding was not an option.

This was integration. And it was a lot more than I had anticipated.

No-one tells you how healing feels like falling apart. I guess you wouldn't believe them if they tried.

I had committed to one MDMA session with Julia out of curiosity, without any expectation about the next steps.

Despite how hard it was, despite the fact that every day, for weeks on end, something new and difficult would emerge, I knew I wanted more.

PART TWO

The Italian Girl

When I was nine years old, I asked my father what his childhood was like.

We were sitting at the dinner table, which was always a relatively formal affair. Fabric napkins with silver napkin rings and a concerto playing in the background.

Dad would sit at one end of the table, my sister and I in the middle facing each other, my mother at the other end.

My father was particular about dinner. He would walk up to the table, which was laden with food, scan the offerings and look up at my mother. 'No potatoes?' he would ask if he couldn't see any, less of a genuine question than an accusation. My mother would answer the question with a cold, 'No,' and then throw him a resentful stare, which he would often miss as he was busy flavouring his steak with mustard.

At the end he would give the meal a mark out of ten – Mum never got more than an 8.5, even with potatoes – then get up and go back to his study.

The conversation at the dinner table would start with Dad asking us what we'd learned at school that day. We'd tell him about handwriting lessons and how we were progressing with our times tables.

But within a minute or so, his attention would drift towards the music and then he would be gone, inside his own head, swept into international maritime case law swirling to the tunes of Mahler.

It was during one of these dinners, as I watched him pushing peas onto his fork with a knife, that I had the urgent desire to know him better. To know what he'd been like at my age.

I just asked the question straight out, like I'd seen Michael Parkinson do on the TV.

'Dad, what was your childhood like?'

He looked up at me, surprised out of his train of thought, and it was clear the interruption didn't please him. His brow furrowed. I'm not sure I'd ever asked him such a direct and personal question.

'It was fine. I generally got on with my brothers.'

'Were you happy?' I probed.

'I think I was, yes.'

I knew the facts of my father's childhood, but none of the substance.

He was the eldest of seven, five boys and two girls. Born the day Prince Charles was born in 1948, a moment of huge celebration in Australia, a country still so desperately attached to its flunky status in the British Commonwealth.

My father was born into a well-educated, Anglican family, its family tree dotted with lawyers and clergymen. Wealthy, too. The company my great-grandfather founded in 1934 is one of Australia's longest privately owned family businesses.

Mum told me Dad grew up fat, shy and bullied at school. As she described it, he had an avuncular but busy father and an emotionally distant mother who had herself been raised by an emotionally distant mother.

He'd found validation at school when the teachers figured out that he was bright and hardworking. That was the genesis of his workaholism, Mum said, that he could get attention and love if he excelled academically.

Dad agreed with the fat and bullied bit. The rest of the story he contested, and I watched my parents argue about it on more than one occasion.

The only childhood story he ever shared with me was the one where he received the highest mark in a primary school history essay and the teacher praised him in front of the class.

Perhaps his tormentors, the boys who laughed at his weight and lack of athletic skill, were in the room to hear it.

He told me that story more than once, and in retelling it, his face would light up, almost as if he was a child sharing the best part of his day with an attentive parent.

The quality of Dad's upbringing was a mystery to me, but not my mother's. I can't remember a time when I didn't know how much she hated her father and how much she wanted to be closer to her mother.

The details of my mother's sad and violent childhood were so vivid for me that her stories took up more room in my head than those of my own childhood. I could retell them as if I'd been there.

Mum was an only child of poor, uneducated Italian immigrants. Mum used to say they were middle class, but that was a stretch. Her father and grandfather came here with very little money and moved straight to north Queensland, where they lived in tin sheds and worked their guts out in the heat and the humidity, the rats and the spiders, cutting sugar cane for months on end.

They saved up and bought farmland and then cut cane for themselves. Brought over more relatives, who would cook in the farm kitchens if they were women, cut cane if they were men.

I wrote a book about my mother's origins, *The Italian Girl*. Part memoir, part history, a love letter to the women in my family. It was ostensibly about my mother's mother. About what happened when the men were interned as enemy aliens during the Second World War.

My nonna, in her twenties with minimal English and no formal education beyond primary school, was left to run the cane farms for years while they waited for the men to be released.

The book was an attempt to understand my grandmother as a young woman, before she became the gentle, diligent homemaker I knew growing up. Her hidden capacities and strengths; her thwarted desires.

The book ends at the point my mother is born in 1945, a few months after the end of the war in the Pacific.

My mother was the only daughter of first cousins. Not uncommon in those days, when migrant families were so tight-knit and isolated from the broader community, daughters sequestered to the home and chaperoned at all times.

Nonna was the youngest of seven, and by the time her father, Luigi, was interned the family was running a number of farms and doing well.

My nonno, however, was the only son of Luigi's sister, and their family was genuinely poor. My nonno's father was an eccentric, half-in-the-closet gay man with a penchant for opera and lace tablecloths. Nonno's mother was a sad, worn, humiliated woman. She stayed in Italy with her only other child, a spinster daughter, and didn't migrate with the rest of the family.

Poverty and shame had made my nonno resentful and taciturn, a man whose only real satisfaction in life had been playing soccer.

He had a violent temper, and it turns out its main target was my mother.

Mum told me her earliest memory was experiencing a searing pain in her head and reaching up to feel a warm patch of blood spreading through her hair. She had been slurping her soup at the table. Her father, enraged by the sound, had struck her.

My mother was, like me, an indoor child. North Queensland was full of things that could kill you in theatrical ways. Insane levels of humidity and heat. Cyclones and floods that destroyed properties and killed people. Crocodiles swam in the waters around her home town of Innisfail. Deadly spiders and disease-carrying rats infested every natural environment from the vegetable patch to the cane fields. A local chapter of the Calabrian mafia ran an extortion racket up and down 'the sugar coast'.

Given all this, it seemed wise to keep indoors.

Mum never learned to swim or ride a bicycle. She stayed

in and around her home as a child, and was even tied to the washing line with a rope if her mother needed to venture far without her.

She went to and from Catholic school, taught by a huddle of industrial-strength nuns. If she made a mistake during piano practice, one of the Good Samaritan sisters would stab her offending hand with a knitting needle.

She'd leave home for church on Sundays, of course. A rare excursion into town, where she remembers feeling the uncloaked hostility of the Anglo-Saxon locals. Racism against Italians was intense in the north and widespread in Australia up until the 1970s.

Italian was my mother's first language; she learned English at primary school. She never spoke to me about whispering in class with friends or skipping-ropes in the playground. There were no sleepovers or birthday parties.

Mum was a sickly child. She would be struck down with chest infections on a regular basis. She told me being sick was her only respite from her father's violence. And when she was unwell, her hardworking mother would have to carve out time from running the farm house and cane cutters' kitchen to tend to her.

Sickness meant not only rest, but safety. And attention.

I don't think I can remember a time when my mother hasn't been unwell with something – sinus, asthma, rosacea, chest infections, chronic pain in her knees, and then, in her late sixties, various cancers.

Or just unwell. In a kind of unspecified way.

I can see now that sickness provided a refuge for her, a legitimate excuse to withdraw, to stay in bed with tea and television, cats as her companions. Away from obligations and people.

*

My parents meeting and marrying was an improbable story.

They first encountered each other in a history tutorial at the University of Adelaide in the late 1960s. Mum had re-enrolled in her arts degree after dropping out to travel, determined to finish so she could start work as a teacher. She used to tell me she felt like the only wog on campus. Classmates, when they found out she was Italian, would sneer and ask if her parents ran a fruit and vegetable shop.

The way Mum tells it, when she first laid eyes on Dad he was sitting alone, muttering under his breath after the lecturer had said something he didn't agree with.

My mother's romantic interest in my father was bewildering to me, even when I first heard these stories as a child. All her dating stories prior to meeting him featured football players and racing car drivers. Men who were suave alpha males.

But my father's reputation had preceded him. Other people had told Mum he was brilliant, a hugely attractive quality to a highly intelligent woman whose cleverness was regularly underestimated.

I still don't know how they started talking. They did share a love of history. Perhaps post-lecture chats about the Russian pogroms led to coffee?

Dad had only dated a few women before he met Mum. I suspect that he had never met anyone like her. Olive-skinned, long dark hair, intense stare, both worldly and from another world. Mum had travelled extensively through Europe, whereas Dad had rarely ventured beyond the tight boundaries of Adelaide.

The way she tells it, she had been engaged a few times but had always broken it off – once, a few days before the wedding. She escaped to Italy instead of telling the hapless fellow she had changed her mind, leaving it to my nonna to do the jilting. 'He was devastated,' Mum used to tell me, with only a hint of remorse.

It was Adelaide in the 1960s, so people like my parents didn't live together or date for long before getting married. Dad proposed, and very quickly they organised a simple ceremony at an Anglican church and a breakfast reception with croissants and champagne.

Mum wore an elegant and simple long-sleeved white dress and a veil, her long hair flowing. Dad looked overjoyed in the photos. His family's emotions about the day are less clear. Given the sentiment of the times, they can't have been chuffed that their eldest son had married a poor Roman Catholic girl.

'Did Nonno give you away?' I asked my mother once.

'No, they were in Italy.'

'Your parents didn't see you get married? Why didn't you wait until they got back?'

'I didn't want my father there. I didn't want him to give me away.'

Mum thought she was marrying a man entirely different from her own father: my father was tall, educated, Anglo and wealthy. Not true, of course. Her father and her new husband had a lot in common, but how could she have possibly known that at the time? What looked like an escape was in fact anything but.

Like I said, my parents' union was an improbable one but with a predictable ending.

Kitten goes splat

All divorces are hard, but each divorce is hard in its own way.

My parents' divorce was a series of shocks and increasingly bizarre scenes that led to my father walking out the front door and disappearing for years.

By the time I hit thirteen, after several tumultuous years moving between Sydney, Oxford, Cambridge and Adelaide, we were back in Sydney. This time for good, apparently.

Sydney would provide status for Dad, and stability for the rest of us. He'd been given a chair in international law at the University of Sydney. Mum would return to part-time teaching. I'd go to the local high school, Emily back to the primary school we'd attended during our last Sydney stint.

Dad had been flying to and from Sydney for some time for work, but also to find us a place to live. After months of searching, he found a beautiful house with a swimming pool in a cul-de-sac in Sydney's eastern suburbs, a short bus ride from my new school.

The thought of being able to swim every day to lose weight had its appeal, but still, I didn't want to move again.

Since moving back to Adelaide, I'd been attending a private school where my mother worked. Instead of beginning high school with all the other students, I had arrived mid-year so Dad could have his sabbatical in Cambridge.

As the new girl, I had endured months of merciless bullying for my weight, my bad skin, my out-of-control hair and my awkward demeanour.

I was a strange mix of horribly self-conscious and intellectually snobbish. By the time I was twelve, I'd read Homer, Jane Austen and George Orwell. I'd seen more operas than pop music concerts.

I was a weirdo.

After the new-girl hazing subsided and I'd ingested enough *Dolly* magazine to fit in with my peers, I managed to settle into a friendship group. I was happy and doing well at school. I didn't want to have to start again.

As the time approached for us to leave Adelaide, I pooled my pocket money to buy small gifts for all the girls in my class. Scented erasers and stickers. Things thirteen-year-old girls in my day loved to collect. I wrapped each meticulously and hid them under my bed in a cardboard box.

Something – some instinct that this gesture would upset my parents – made me hide the gifts.

My sister discovered them and told my parents.

Dad was furious. He stormed into the room, pulled the gifts out from under my bed and started throwing them on the floor one by one. My mother watched silently from the adjoining room, my sister a few steps behind her, looking stricken.

He shouted about my ungrateful behaviour, accusing me of only caring about my friends and not my family.

He grabbed me by the shoulder with one hand and held one of the little packages up to my face with the other.

'You are buying gifts for your friends while I'm slaving away to buy a house with a swimming pool so you don't get fatter than you already are.'

He let go of me, tossed the gift on the floor and pounded down the hallway towards his bedroom. Emily had disappeared. Mum glanced at me with a mixture of fatigue and annoyance and went to check on my father.

I gathered up all the gifts, rewrapped the ones that had been torn in my father's rampage, and stashed them in a better hiding place.

This was the first time I remember feeling that my father's rage was unjustified, his words unnecessarily cruel, my mother's bystander stance a betrayal.

I was beginning, just a little, to doubt my parents' notions of wisdom and justice.

*

Their marriage started to disintegrate the year after we moved back to Sydney, and I began to truly comprehend the emotional chaos of our lives.

I could feel things were falling apart. Mum was tired all the time, and seemed happiest in her bedroom alone. Dad was increasingly absent, and when he was around there was a new kind of strained energy between them.

One evening as I was sitting in my room doing homework, the door flung open and my mother walked in.

'I need you in the bedroom.'

Everything about my mother at that moment – her face, her body movements, her tone of voice – told me this was not 'I need you in the bedroom cos you're getting a pony.'

It was 'I need you in the bedroom so we can pour some gasoline on this bin-fire of a family.'

With a heavy heart, I made my way to the front of the house.

My sister was sitting on the end of my parents' bed, wide-eyed and pale. My father sat in a chair in the corner of the room with a look I'd never seen before, one of abject shame. Mum crawled into bed and under the covers.

'Tell them what you just told me.'

My father looked at her pleadingly. Again, something new to me.

'Please don't.'

'Tell them.'

He looked at my sister and me and said, *sotto voce*, 'I slept with …' He named a female colleague of his.

I knew her name because I had teased him about her, saying she had a crush on him. He'd had more than a few dinners with her over the previous months. 'Seems like you are off on a date, Dad,' I said one time as he was walking out the door to meet her. He smirked and said nothing.

Something inside me crumpled when my father said those words. I knew it at the time, could name it. It was the collapse of my belief that everything my father did, all his hours at work and his monumental stress that would explode into anger every few weeks, was for our benefit. To provide for us.

That if he had any spare time on his hands, it would be spent with us.

A huge chunk of my love and almost all of my respect for my father evaporated in that moment, as I sat on my mother's bed watching him shrink into the chair.

It was a con job. All of it. He wasn't slaving away so I could live in a nice house with a pool so I wouldn't get fatter. He was slaving away so he could feel important and loved and have sex with other women.

All of a sudden, he looked small to me, sitting in that chair. And as a result, I was less afraid of him.

Which meant I felt free to yell at him, for the first time in my life. 'How could you?' or something akin to that, and then I ran out of the room, only to be told to return, somewhat angrily, by my mother.

Perhaps she wanted me to stay by her side so I could yell at him some more.

An outburst of this kind would normally be met with a disproportionate response.

Instead, my father did nothing.

Whatever happened or was said next, I can't remember. But I do remember it was the last time for a long time we'd all be in a room together.

*

A couple of months after Dad's confession, I got my first job. I had turned fourteen and was old enough to be paid cash in hand as a filing girl at a doctors' office. The office was in Paddington, one of Sydney's more exclusive suburbs. The doctors were fancy and so were the clients. I would take a bus there after school and spend a few hours putting patients' paper files back in their proper order.

One of the doctors had a kind of registered sex offender vibe. I gave him a nickname, Dr Smarm. The woman running the reception was the main doctor's second wife, and she looked like an off-brand backup singer from a Robert Palmer video. All red lipstick, tight black clothes and slicked-back hair. She was addicted to filing her nails, rather than filing. So, they paid my friend Wendy and me to job share. Ten dollars an hour – a lot in those days.

In the middle of all the tumult at home, this felt like freedom. A job and my own money. I think I blew my first pay packet on clothes.

After Dad had disclosed his affair, my parents had entered a 'let's try to resuscitate our relationship' phase.

Dad moved out to a little terrace house a few suburbs away, a trial separation while they worked on their marriage. They were going to start dating again and see a couples' therapist.

This new halfway house of Dad's was equidistant from the family home and his lover's house in Paddington. My sister and I had one meal at his new digs and saw that they were suspiciously clean, which made me wonder how much time he was spending there outside the office.

My parents attended a few sessions of therapy until it started to clash with Dad's work commitments. Their dates were few and far between.

A woman would call the house late at night looking for him, sounding desperate, upset or drunk – it was hard for a teenager to tell. She would ask in a slurred voice if she could please speak to him. 'Dad doesn't live here at the moment,' I'd say, and put down the receiver without waiting for a reply.

Without my father, our house felt calmer. Gone was that ever-present edginess I felt, waiting for the next work-triggered eruption.

But with Dad no longer living there, my mother's moods were free to expand, to take up all the space available. She was up and down, desolate one moment, apoplectically angry the next, with occasional bursts of euphoria.

A few days after the confrontation in the bedroom, Mum came home from a doctor's appointment suspiciously upbeat and smiling. 'The doctor told me Dad's problems can be cured. There's a solution. He's depressed. There are pills for that. It's going to be okay.' She hugged me and practically skipped up the hallway to her bedroom.

Her excitement exhausted me. I knew their marriage was over, even if she didn't.

My sister and I watched my mother's moods closely and adapted to each swing.

We kept going to school, did what we could around the house, kept our grades up.

We ate a lot of takeaway pizza.

Dad was still turning up at the house occasionally. Sometimes he arrived before we woke up. Other times, we would hear his voice late at night.

Whenever he visited, my parents would inevitably fight. One time, his arrival coincided with our return from yet another Pizza Hut run. Dad said something and Mum hit him with a family-sized Supreme. The pizza flew out of the box and hit the grass, topping-side up.

After Dad fled and Mum went inside, my sister and I retrieved the pizza from the lawn and picked out the blades of grass so we could eat it.

I started to cook more after that.

There were times when I had to get Mum out of bed, take off her nightgown, put her in the shower, take her out and dry her down, then dress her again. It was as if she was sleepwalking, eyes fixed on some unknown object in the distance.

Emily spent a lot of time alone in her room, disappearing into her favourite books and TV shows.

I wish I could say I made sure she was okay.

*

My friends, my school, my new job. These were my own private escapes.

One of my first afternoons working at the doctor's surgery, I was silently cycling the alphabet through my head as I wedged large and small files into the shelves next to the receptionist table when the door flew open.

It was a tiny reception area. Three large strides and you could move from the seats by the window and be at the desk to sign your receipt.

I turned to see my mother at the threshold. The abrupt noise of the door flinging open had startled all the people in the waiting room – the patients leafing through magazines, Robert Palmer's backup singer and Dr Smarm, who was exiting his office with a patient.

I walked briskly over to my mother to ask her what was wrong. 'Rebecca, you need to come with me right now,' my mother said in a voice bristling with anger. 'He's with her, he's at her house.'

I knew who the 'he' and the 'her' were without being told. The doctors' office was in the same suburb my father's lover lived in.

I told my mum I felt bad about leaving work.

'You need to leave and come with me now.'

I turned to my employers and offered a somewhat rushed apology, promising I'd either come back later or work more hours the next day. Dr Smarm gave me a disapproving look as we left.

We got into Mum's car and drove for a few minutes, to a modest little terrace in a tree-lined street. Mum had been there once for a dinner party the year before. Maybe she had driven past it a few times since, to check it out. She was certainly convinced Dad was there now.

Part of me thought Mum was being paranoid, but when we arrived, his distinctive yellow Volvo with familiar plates was parked outside the house.

It was the middle of the afternoon on a work day. The dad I knew barely paused to take a toilet break in the middle of the afternoon on a work day.

We sat parked across the street in silence. Mum was staring at the door. I looked at her, at her beautiful profile. She hated her nose. It was prominent. But she looked like one of those women you see in ancient frescos in Italian villas. Bewitching. Regal. Dangerous.

'Go and knock on the door and tell him to come out,' Mum told me.

I keep returning to this moment, trying to remember how this fourteen-year-old girl, who wanted to be back at work, felt when her mother insisted that she interrupt her father fucking his lover.

I can't remember how I felt. I only remember I did it without demurring, because to say no was unthinkable.

I got out, crossed the street and walked up to the solid wooden door. I knocked, then waited. Nothing. I knocked again, a little louder.

'Dad, it's Rebecca, can you come out please?' I tried to block out all thoughts about what was happening on the other side of that solid door.

Still no word. I heard footsteps behind the door, then silence.

I went back to sit in the car with Mum.

'He's not coming out.'

She handed me her extra key to the Volvo.

'Go see if his wallet and his briefcase are inside the car. Take them and bring them back here. We will go to his office and wait.'

*

As a teenager I used to jokingly tell my friends that my father was born in a suit. I think I saw him in jeans once, when he had to take a trip to Arnhem Land to consult with First Nations groups about customary law. Other than that brief spell in informal wear, he dressed like he was working at a law firm rather than a law school. His tastes were highbrow, too. German opera, French food and English antiques. He was, even in his late thirties, revered and probably a little resented by his colleagues.

He had a big city office in the law school tower near the courts. I'd been there a few times. I'm not sure I'd ever been there with my mother, though, so when we walked in carrying his briefcase, without an appointment, his secretary must have been perplexed.

She ushered us into his office and Mum and I sat on the couch facing his desk to await his inevitable arrival.

It didn't take long for Dad to turn up. He walked in without even glancing in our direction, less flustered than he should have been, in my view, went to his desk and started shuffling papers as if he was alone in the room.

Mum sat, arms crossed, staring at him with contempt.

After a few seconds of strange silence, I spoke first.

'Dad, why didn't you open the door?'

He looked up at me and said coldly, 'I don't open the door to crazy people.'

Well, that was it.

I gave it to the Challis Professor of whatever with both barrels.

I yelled at my father like I had never yelled at anyone in my life.

I can't recall exactly what I said, but I remember the major themes. His disrespect for Mum. His weakness. His betrayal.

Dad was clearly taken aback by my outburst, but instead of responding, he took off down the corridor.

'He's probably gone to his car,' Mum said calmly. 'Go after him.'

I dutifully followed him.

His office was on one of the higher floors. I just missed him getting into the lift, and so I ran down the fire stairs at speed.

The lift must have stopped at a few floors on its trajectory towards the basement because I entered the car park just as he was about to get into his car.

I ran to stand in front of the Volvo so he couldn't escape. I continued to berate him.

The lies, the betrayal. Mum wasn't mad. I wasn't mad. He was the mad one.

The basement of the law school was quite small and reserved only for the most important of the academics. The exit fronted onto a major CBD street with a bus stop, so students would often take a shortcut through the basement to get to the lifts rather than lug their heavy books up the stairs to the main foyer.

I became aware of a steady stream of students passing by only a few metres away.

I turned to them, pointed at my father and shouted, 'Look! Look at this man you think is so great. He's not. He's a liar. All he does is lie.'

The students appeared only marginally less embarrassed than my father.

I must have scared everyone away, because within a few seconds we were alone.

My father had been speechless and almost motionless during this scene. His face had the same kind of shameful look as the one he had sported when he'd revealed his infidelity.

The car door was open but he still hadn't gotten in. Both arms were on the hood of his car and he was clinging to it like a life raft as his teenage daughter vented her rage towards him in the place where his authority usually went unchallenged.

Finally, I was all yelled out.

Then I said softly, 'You hit me, Dad. You hit me a lot. My whole life. You hit me.'

Throughout this encounter my father's head was slightly bowed, but in response to my words he straightened up, let go of the car, looked me squarely in the face and replied, with absolute certainty, 'I never laid a hand on you.'

At that moment, I felt a sense of release. Not the crumpling I'd experienced in my parents' bedroom at the admission of the affair, but a realisation that if Dad could deny ever raising his hand to me, it would be impossible to have an honest conversation with him. About anything. Probably ever.

I let go of any hope that he could ever be a father to me. Hope would mean expectation, and expectation would mean disappointment.

I turned around to see my mother watching from near the lift doors. There it was. Her usual impassive face, but something subtle in the lift of her brow. Triumph, maybe?

'Let's go home, Rebecca.'

She'd parked in one of the few car spots reserved for visitors. We got into our second-hand Toyota Corolla and drove away. My father stood and watched us leave.

*

Movie scenes where the protagonist confronts the person who wronged them in public are usually jubilant and cathartic. Worthy of a stirring soundtrack. Close-ups. People standing on tables, etc.

There was nothing cathartic about yelling at Dad in the law school basement. I felt some satisfaction that I had stood up to my father for my mother's sake, but I also felt deflated. I knew I had to fashion new truths to live by out of the wreck of my parents' marriage and the disintegration of my family. But I had no idea how to do that.

I saw Dad one last time during this period, a few weeks after the incident in the law school basement.

I remember it well because he threw a kitten at me.

I woke up to yelling in the kitchen one morning, and emerged to see my mother and father screaming at each other. He was in the lounge room and she was in the kitchen.

Dad had never hit Mum. Not in front of me and not behind closed doors, to my knowledge.

Mum had confided in me that he had tried to do so once. A few weeks after their wedding, Mum had told my father she'd made a mistake marrying him. That had caused a heated argument between them and she said that at one point Dad went to strike her across the face. She took an empty beer bottle, smashed it on the side of the kitchen counter and, as blood ran down her hands, raised the broken glass towards him and told him if he ever touched her in anger, she would kill him.

While I took this story with a grain of salt, I could imagine it happening. That it was something she was capable of doing. That he was capable of that kind of violence in the face of rejection.

But at this moment, as they were screaming at each other in front of me, I had an inkling that he wanted to hit her.

I knew the signs that he was about to lash out too well. The wild sweating face, his voice going up an octave, the way his words started to bleed into one long sentence, so different from the measured tones in which he would lecture students or talk to dinner party guests.

But then he did something unexpected. He started hitting himself, bashing his temple with his fist. Once. Then a few more times. A small gash started to appear. Then some blood.

I watched him for a few seconds, startled. He seemed to have gone completely mad, to hit himself in the head like that. As children we were told to never touch my father's head, even playfully. 'What's in his head is precious, Rebecca,' my mother used to say. I recall the few times I'd accidentally touched his face how he would aggressively flinch and recoil. And yet here he was smashing his priceless head over and over.

I realised some significant shift in my attitude towards my father had occurred because instead of being scared or worried, I found myself thinking, *Do us all a favour and knock yourself out, you arsehole.*

The blood stopped them fighting, and my mother went to get my father a towel to stem the bleeding. He took it, shoving off her attempts to help him, and then he turned and headed down the hallway towards their bedroom.

The last dregs of filial concern must have been what led me down the hall to see if Dad was alright, or still in the house.

As part of his half-hearted attempts to placate my mother when the affair was first disclosed, he'd bought her two

Burmese kittens. Mum's previous beloved Burmese Sophie had died, run over during our first stay in Sydney. My mother grieved hard when that cat was killed; Sophie had been her only real friend during that time. Dad thought he could placate her with the same kind of cat twice over. One of the kittens he had sourced was the runt of the litter, a tiny brown thing we named Georgia.

Georgia practically lived on my mother's bed, and as I stood in the hallway and peered into their room, I could see my father sitting on the edge of the bed, the picture of total dejection. He was clutching Georgia – perhaps for some kind of comfort – with one hand, and holding the towel against his forehead with the other.

'Dad, are you okay?'

He looked up at me. And then he threw the kitten.

Dad was a massive cricket fan. He fancied himself a spin bowler but was notoriously bad at it – which was good news for the kitten. She hit the wall without much force, slid down it, lay there for a split second, then shook herself and got the hell out of Dodge. (She survived, but she walked with a kink in her step for the rest of her life.)

You never forget the sound, the soft thunk, of your father throwing a kitten at you. And with that final gesture, he walked out the door, for all I knew never to be seen again.

*

A few weeks after the kitten-throwing incident, removalists turned up to take away my father's family heirlooms.

Three grim portraits of Scottish ancestors, which would not be missed. And a grandfather clock, which I loved. Its sonorous, hourly chime always signalled that I'd done enough maths homework.

Then: nothing.

No word from my father. For years.

Of course, he was still in Sydney and so were we. I spent a lot of time in the CBD near the law school and he walked past me a few times, but I can't be sure he saw me.

One time, though, he definitely did. I was sitting on the law school steps waiting for a bus, just a few metres away from the infamous basement.

I turned to see the nose of his yellow Volvo poking out of the exit, just as he turned his head towards me. He saw me. A second passed. Then he looked away.

A few months after that sighting I got my final exam results. I did well, but not well enough to get into law school straight from high school. The threshold was 98.25 and I got 98.2.

That was a high mark. It put me in the top 1.8 per cent of the state, but there was no celebration.

Mum was bitterly disappointed. She wanted me to be in the top one per cent of the state. My whole life she told me how clever I was. Cleverer than my father. 'You know children get their intelligence from the maternal line. Never forget that,' she would say.

A week or so after I got my disappointing results, I heard from Dad. A card arrived in the mail. The final exam marks of every student in the state were published in the newspaper. Perhaps he'd had a look.

Cards are nice, but I'd also been hoping for a cheque or something.

I opened the card, addressed to me in his distinctive cursive handwriting. The front of the card was white and gold, embossed with flowers. *Deepest condolences*, it said.

My father had accidentally put the wrong card in the wrong envelope. Somewhere, some widow would receive a 'Congratulations on finishing your exams' card, with a $100 gift voucher to David Jones.

But I was wrong. It was the right card. Inside, he had crossed out the schmaltzy Hallmark poem about loss and written:

Dear Rebecca

So near and yet so far.

Dad

Then a year or so later at breakfast, we opened the newspaper to see a large photo of my father and an extensive article. He'd been appointed to the prestigious international law chair at Cambridge University. Not Oxford as he had wanted, but Cambridge. Nevertheless, it was the next crucial rung on the ladder towards the International Court of Justice, and greatness.

Mum peered over my shoulder and we read the article together.

'Perhaps you need to get in contact and see him before he goes.'

I can't recall what the article said, but my sister remembers one particular comment he made: that it was time to leave Australia. That there was nothing keeping him here.

I did as Mum had suggested and contacted Dad at the law school. He suggested dinner at the Opera House. I was twenty and in my first year of law school – not the one he had presided over, but another. I made my boyfriend tag along.

It was less awkward than it could have been. We talked about his work, and my study. By then I excelled at small talk. I'd had a lifetime of practice pretending everything was okay.

But underneath the smiles and questions about Cambridge, I was angry. I didn't give a damn about his brilliant career, because I was its collateral damage.

Session two

It was a surprise to me that my father's violence and the laughably horrible scenes of my parents' divorce didn't feature more prominently in my first session on MDMA. In the final hours of the session, I did talk at length to Julia about my father and how his abuse and then abandonment made me feel.

But when the drug had its firmest hold on me, what I remembered, and re-remembered, were scenes of significance for me as a mother, as my mother's daughter, as a sister. Of love, but also of failure. My failure to protect and care for Emily.

Julia kept telling me the drug knew what it was doing. The drug has its own 'wisdom', she said, more than once.

Although some of them felt puzzling to me, the memories MDMA made me recall and relive were, in fact, exactly what I needed to recall and relive in order to heal.

In the aftermath of the first session, I became more curious about the drug and the process I'd signed up for.

I read some of the peer-reviewed journal articles on MDMA therapy, which described the medical research in detail. With the Australian Therapeutic Goods Administration decision to allow psychiatrists to prescribe to the public, the outcomes of the clinical trials were being scrutinised across the media.

People were describing MDMA therapy as a 'potential breakthrough' for people with post-traumatic stress disorder who were finding conventional treatments ineffective. Conventional treatments meaning talk therapy, but also drugs, including selective serotonin reuptake inhibitors (SSRIs) like Lexapro, Zoloft and Prozac.

Formal research on MDMA had stalled during its criminalisation, but thanks to the indefatigable efforts of the US-based organisation MAPS, this had started up again.

The most widely talked about research was a randomised, double blind, placebo-controlled study involving ninety patients. They received therapy with MDMA or with a placebo, combined with three sessions before and nine sessions after with a therapist.

They found that MDMA therapy was 'highly efficacious in individuals with severe PTSD'.

The researchers theorised that MDMA was so effective

because it can 'reopen an oxytocin-dependent critical period of neuroplasticity that typically closes after adolescence'.

This then allows for the processing and release of particular fear-based memories. Because the drug subdues the amygdala, preventing the patient from becoming overwhelmed by emotions, it can produce a 'window of tolerance', allowing the patient to revisit and process traumatic experiences without becoming highly reactive or disassociating.[13]

The literature on these trials reinforced what Julia had been telling me since the beginning. The substance itself, while powerful, doesn't work effectively on its own. It can accelerate healing. But without the hours of therapy before and after with specially trained professionals, it's just a drug.

Of course, the media reports on the legalisation of MDMA therapy focused on just the drug, the stigma around it and its more common recreational use. They often failed to mention one of the main reasons why further research into MDMA is desperately needed: because the usual drugs being prescribed to treat mental illness are not working as well as we'd like them to. These drugs – namely SSRIs – have high failure rates when taken for either mild depression or more extreme conditions like PTSD. Rates of anywhere between forty and sixty per cent, depending on how you measure failure.[14]

Despite these high failure rates, we keep on taking them, in greater numbers with each passing year. More Australians are taking antidepressants and anti-anxiety medications than ever before, with prescription rates doubling over the past ten years. Australia has the second-highest per capita usage of antidepressants of all OECD countries, following Iceland.[15]

All around the world, prescriptions for these medications are rising exponentially. The global pandemic saw a bump in already high levels of people taking prescription drugs for anxiety and depression in countries like the US, the UK, Canada, Sweden, Spain and Germany, as well as Australia.[16]

And there are few signs that, now the pandemic is 'over', these levels will fall. Indeed, there is evidence that, post-pandemic, in countries where SSRI intake is already high, depression and anxiety are continuing to climb.[17]

The medical researchers responsible for the ninety-person clinical trial wrote that in countries like Australia and around the world, we are facing a double whammy when it comes to mental health. We have more people with depression, anxiety, PTSD and other chronic mental health issues, and we have inadequate or limited tools and resources to deal with them. They wrote:

> *We may soon be confronted with the potentially enormous economic and social repercussions of PTSD, exacerbated by the COVID-19 pandemic. Overwhelmingly high rates of*

> *psychological and mental health impairment could be with us for years to come and are likely to impart a considerable emotional and economic burden.*[18]

Drugs like SSRIs have their use. They can be life-changing, live-saving solutions for people who are suffering.

But increasingly, people in the medical profession, everyone from local doctors to eminent psychologists and psychiatrists, are pointing out that there is an alarming over-reliance on these drugs.[19]

In my life I've known too many people whose complex childhood trauma manifests as anxiety or depression later in life. They see a doctor who may or may not ask the right questions, after making sure there is no immediate risk of self-harm. They walk out half an hour or so later with a prescription and a referral to a therapist.

There is rarely any follow-up about whether they have in fact found a therapist and if they are going regularly or just shuffling in and out (like I did for years).

Certainly, the drugs are far cheaper and more accessible than the therapy. Repeat prescriptions are pretty easy to get. Or they might shop around to various GPs so they can continue with the drugs that keep their worst symptoms in check. One drug stops working as well, so they try another.

The drugs help them not to feel so sad, so anxious, help them sleep, help them get out of bed. Go to work. Be a reasonably productive, law-abiding taxpayer.

They don't feel as bad as they did before the drugs because they mostly feel numb. The lows are gone but so are the highs. Including in some cases sexual desire. No despair, but also no joy.

For the many people I know who have gone down this path of prescription medication and stop-start therapy, it can stretch on for years, decades even.

It's like keeping a lid on a boiling pot without turning the heat down.

To be clear, this isn't me masking my own personal experience. I was on SSRIs once, for about six months in my mid-twenties, to address my fear of flying. In conjunction with the cognitive behavioural therapy, the drugs worked so well that I left a dysfunctional relationship and finished my doctorate on time, the two pressing reasons I'd been feeling so shitty. For me, the antidepressants were a firm outstretched hand helping me up off the floor. But that stint on the drug and with the therapist didn't even begin to address the root cause of my problems.

Now that I was in the middle of this different kind of drug therapy, I wondered how effective just talking about my problems had been. Wondered how long going to Karen once a month and my regular self-regulating activities – exercise in nature and time with friends – would have taken to get me to the point where I found myself after only one MDMA session.

Could I have reached it without the drug and Julia's psyche midwifery? Maybe.

But what personal suffering did I avoid by getting there faster? And what collateral damage to others has been avoided too?

*

Normally, Julia suggested waiting about two months between sessions.

I understood why. It wasn't just in the few days after the first session that I would be stopped in my tracks by a resurfaced memory. It went on for weeks. I would be sideswiped by a sudden revelation while grocery shopping. I'd review a cherished moment from a different angle in a way that would make me burst into tears as I prepared sandwiches for my kids' lunch. I cried about things that had happened decades ago in a way I hadn't let myself cry at the time.

I marvelled at the impact just one session had on my self-knowledge and my perspective on past hurts. But I worried about how potentially damaging this process could be if you weren't safe, supported, ready for the onslaught of emotions.

And lucky. I was lucky to have decades of therapy behind me, the support of dear friends and my sister, good physical health and no real financial worries.

Even given all that good fortune, I wondered if I was really ready, if I could handle this wisdom the drug was dishing out to me. There were times when I felt like the only thing keeping me from unspooling was having to hold it together for the girls.

Still, I wanted more, and soon.

*

Julia had decided to leave Australia for some time to treat patients in other countries. I wanted a second session before she left, and so she agreed to see me again six weeks after our first session. This time, she would host me in her home.

She lived in a stunningly beautiful, semi-tropical area in the northern part of New South Wales, where three rivers run. The region is something of a hub for people leading alternative lifestyles and, due to some vaccination scepticism, a hotspot for the resurgence of old diseases like diphtheria and whooping cough.

I packed a few masks and a heap of COVID tests in an overnight bag and on a Monday morning in March 2023 took the short flight from Sydney to Ballina, the airport closest to Julia's home. I booked accommodation nestled into the side of a mountain in the Byron Bay Hinterland. Google Maps told me it was only a fifteen-minute drive down the mountain to Julia.

The flight was delayed, so I arrived in Ballina late. A car service drove me through the leafy outer suburbs of the town, up the mountain and dropped me at my accommodation. It had a beautiful pool with a panoramic view of the bush and the ocean. I'd splurged on the place. If things were going to get emotionally messy, I wanted to fall apart in Egyptian cotton sheets.

I was served a meal in my room. Afterwards, as I lay in bed waiting to fall asleep, I wondered whether the drug would work as well a second time, and if it did, where it would take me.

I was due at Julia's after 10 am the next day. I didn't need to rush, but I woke at 6 am regardless. It was hot and humid, even before breakfast. I swam in the pool and drank in the view of the trees and the water.

I followed Julia's instructions to avoid stimulants like coffee, and so I drank herbal tea.

I asked the accommodation manager when I should set off, given I would be on foot. I gave her the address.

'That's a big walk down the mountain and along the roadside.'

'I like walking.'

'I could organise a taxi, but they don't really like to come up here unless they are taking people to the airport. Maybe a car service? The one that dropped you off would do it.'

'I'm fine. I like walking.'

She nodded and gave me a 'suit yourself' smile. 'If I was you, I'd head off now before it gets really hot. Take it slow.'

I find asking for help extremely difficult. If anyone ever says, 'It looks like you need help,' I immediately get annoyed. What I really hear them saying is, 'It looks like you can't cope. You look weak. Vulnerable. And if you are weak and vulnerable and need help, that's your fault. You didn't plan. You weren't smart enough. You are selfish because you didn't have a smart plan and now you are asking for help.'

I'd talked to Karen about this aversion to asking for help. Or, more accurately, she'd talked to me about it. I couldn't see the problem myself. I was resourceful. Flexible. Strong. This was a part of me that I cherished so much that I thought it deserved its own tattoo, which I had needled onto my right wrist during my fiftieth year: 22TI. In the periodic table that's the symbol for titanium, the metal with the highest strength-to-flexibility ratio.

I felt a protective pride about this part of me, but Karen gave it a label that made me feel less pleased with myself. She called it hyper-independence. I googled it. A classic coping mechanism for people with experience of complex childhood trauma. Duh.

Julia had offered to pick me up from my accommodation and drive me home at the end of the session. The drive home I reluctantly accepted, as I knew that, post-trip, I'd need some help to get back to the retreat. But I told Julia I'd meet her at her house in the morning.

'I am happy to pick you up. I'm heading out to the markets after breakfast and I can swing by after.'

'It's fine. I like to walk.'

I set off down the mountain at nine. The sun was climbing, and when it broke through the shade with its pounding heat, I took a swig from my water bottle.

The road wasn't built for walking. Bitumen, barely wide enough for two cars and sloping down to deep ditches on both sides to accommodate the rivers of water that would flow during the heavy rains the region was famous for. But I was feeling buoyant. The road was quiet and shaded by eucalyptus and other trees I didn't recognise. Occasionally, a car would make its way past me, the driver giving me a nod. I passed expensive new-looking houses, probably holiday houses or retirement living for city folk. Then dilapidated shacks with rambling veggie gardens and Tibetan prayer flags strung across the porch. Locals.

After ten or so minutes of walking downhill in quiet contemplation and shade, I reached an intersection where the narrow road met a wider two-lane road, flat and stretching for what looked like ages to my left. I checked Google Maps. The road to Julia's place branched off somewhere out of sight. There was no shade to speak of, and I regretted my last-minute decision not to bring a hat. I drained my water bottle and set off.

I trudged along the road feeling stupid, the high spirits of the downhill walk gone. I wondered if I had the chutzpah to flag down a passing car and ask for a lift a few kilometres up the road, closer to Julia. Mobile phone reception was patchy. Even if I wanted to google the number of a car service, I couldn't.

After ten minutes of walking in the unrelenting heat and humidity, experiencing caffeine withdrawals and with nothing in my stomach since 7 pm the night before, I was feeling dizzy. Drenched in sweat with a headache that felt like a rope slowly tightening around my skull, I was mildly panicking. I'd stop and wipe the sweat out of my eyes and check the map. Still at least fifteen minutes' walk. There was nowhere to sit, no cars on the road. Could I knock on the door of the next house I saw, ask for a glass of water and some help? One of the places with the Tibetan prayer flags, maybe?

I felt this was one of the few places in Australia where people might understand what I was doing.

Mobile reception was bad, but I could still message Julia on Signal. After five more minutes of walking, my mild panic deepened to concern. If I arrived heat exhausted with a headache, Julia might postpone the treatment.

I saw a school up ahead. I messaged Julia and asked her to pick me up there. She said she'd see me in ten minutes.

I found a shaded seat near the principal's office and waited to be rescued. I was relieved, but also self-conscious. Did I look like a predator? A vagrant hoping to steal office supplies? A teacher walked past and I flagged her down.

'Excuse me, but I wondered if it's okay if I just sit here out of the sun? I'm visiting a friend and I thought I'd walk to her place, but I underestimated the distance and the heat. She's picking me up here in about ten minutes.'

'It's okay,' she said. 'You look like a parent.'

What does a parent look like? Some flushed, benign middle-aged woman in activewear? I guess I fitted the profile.

As promised, Julia pulled up around ten minutes later in a zippy little hatchback. My relief that I was out of the sun and on my way to start the therapy trumped my embarrassment at having put her out. We chatted about nothing much as we made our way up the long stretch of road and down an unsurfaced side road, towards her home and God knows what.

*

Julia had been living and working out of a relatively secluded bungalow overlooking a picturesque vista of trees and hills. We parked underneath the house and made our way up a wooden staircase to the front door. Inside, there was a small galley kitchen and a large sitting room. Her bedroom was behind a closed door next to the bathroom. Tucked in the corner was a day bed covered in cushions with a view of the fields and hills. Outside, through sliding glass doors, was a long wooden verandah.

As soon as we arrived, I rushed to the bathroom to pee, splash my face and neck with cold water and slurp as much as I could from the tap. I wiped myself dry with a hand towel and stared at myself for a few moments in the mirror.

The redness in my face was subsiding but my scalp still ran with perspiration, and I could see my arms had caught too much sun despite the SPF50 I'd slathered on them.

'*In bocca al lupo.*' I said the words quietly to my reflection.

That's what my mother used to say before I had to do an exam or perform in a play. She would write it on cards to me at Christmas and birthdays, too.

It's an Italian saying, one you say when you want to wish someone good luck. It doesn't translate well, but it literally means 'into the wolf's mouth'.

Stare into the wolf's mouth and don't flinch.

You're supposed to respond, '*Crepi il lupo!*' *May the wolf die.*

My father had his own pre-exam rallying cry.

'Once more unto the breach … once more … Or close the wall up with our English dead.'

Henry V.

I laughed softly. Say what you want about my parents, they knew how to prepare me for battle.

I took one more mouthful of water and left the bathroom.

Julia was in the kitchen unpacking her market vegetables. She invited me to take off my shoes and head over to the day bed so we could get started.

I sat cross-legged and lay back on the pillows, still wiping sweat from my forehead with the edges of my T-shirt. There was a welcome breeze coming through the sliding doors.

Julia sat down in a soft armchair opposite me and put a stone vase with a burst of deep red chrysanthemums on the floor next to the day bed.

'I saw these at the markets and they spoke to me. They said, "You need to buy these for Rebecca."'

If I believed in such things, I would have thought Julia was psychic. I love the colour red. Love red flowers. Chrysanthemums, too. Years ago, a Chinese herbalist suggested I drink a red chrysanthemum tea for its anti-inflammatory and healing properties. To help me have another baby.

I watched Julia's now-familiar ritual of starting up the music, lighting a candle, preparing the two doses of the drug and blessing them.

'We give thanks to the sassafras tree …'

I looked out the window. No sassafras tree to be seen. I'd only ever seen them on hikes through Tasmanian forests. Blackheart sassafras, used for wood and not healing. If you chew the leaves, your tongue tingles.

I swallowed the first dose and lay down. Now that I was off the hot road, I was suddenly very tired. I closed my eyes. I had an eye mask next to me but I didn't need it. With my eyes closed, the cool breeze felt cooler, the noise of the bush louder.

I started to worry that I was still too anxious from the events of the morning for the drug to work properly. Maybe it wouldn't work as well as the last time. Maybe being here in this unfamiliar place, I wouldn't be relaxed and open enough to let the drug pull me from the shore into that warm ocean of emotion and memory.

I lay there in silence. At least, this time, I didn't feel like I needed to dust cobwebs or ask Julia about her life.

I was wrong, of course. The drug worked just fine.

Suddenly I was in a hospital bed, not holding Stella like in the first session, but my firstborn girl, Sofia. Her father was beside me, my mother in the chair opposite.

It felt as if the four of us were truly close in that moment. There was a deep, satisfying connection that felt like the happy ending of a children's fairytale. 'One more push and an episiotomy and they all lived happily ever after …'

The silent tears came streaming down my face again, mingling with the last of the sweat from my scalp.

The drug didn't let me stay there in that warmth for long.

I found myself sitting upright in a different hospital bed, sore from a fresh C-section and looking down on two small babies.

Stella had been given to me as soon as she was born, but it wasn't until three days after the birth that I got to hold Sadie. The nurse delivered her, wrapped tightly, to my room and placed her on the bed next to her twin, reunited in a new world of oxygen and light after wrestling inside me for close to nine months.

I was alone, cold, staring at these two tiny bodies wrapped in pink and blue striped blankets.

The same hospital, the same blankets, these bald, wrinkled little daughters coming out of the same body.

But those two moments were like night and day.

So much had changed between that first birth and the last one.

The tears kept coming.

*

I always knew I wanted to be a mother. It's the only thing I have ever been certain about.

Having kids would be my 'do over'. I'd give them the kind of childhood I didn't get to experience. It was a repair fantasy, too. My family was broken even before my parents separated. I'd have children, and through my children I'd create a happier, stronger family, not just for myself but for my sister and my mother. We'd leave the past behind.

As soon as my then-husband, Daniel, and I decided to start trying, I got pregnant. Easy pregnancy. Healthy, easy baby.

My expectation was that being a mother would be hard. Challenging. A huge responsibility, a burden even.

I never expected it to be joyful. To be fun.

When I sat with my baby on my lap, she had the ability to anchor me in the moment. I would just hold her, and for a few minutes I would feel free of the need to be racing forwards or glancing back. The whirligig would stop turning.

When I was first pregnant the plan had been, have one and see how it goes. Perhaps it would be harder than I was expecting. Perhaps I wouldn't be any good at it.

After a year, I couldn't imagine not having more.

All I knew was that I wanted more.

If only life turned out just like you wanted it to.

You have to pay to watch *Law and Order*

After a few minutes wandering the hospital halls, Daniel and I found the office. There were couples sitting in plastic chairs waiting, staff busy with clipboards talking to patients. There are always phones ringing in hospitals; phones that can ring forever because no-one has a spare second to pick them up.

'Excuse me,' I said to a nurse walking past me. I lowered my voice a little. 'I'm here to give birth but, um, not in the usual way.'

She had stopped to smile at me when I said, 'Excuse me,' but as I continued, the smile faded a little and the expression on her face shifted from 'What can I do for you?' to 'What do you mean?'

'The baby's dead. I'm here for an induction.'

Her expression changed quickly again, from confusion to something like tenderness, and she led us – me in a maternity dress and Daniel holding my overnight bag – towards a special suite of rooms.

Three years earlier, almost to the day, I'd been in the same wing of the same hospital giving birth to my daughter Sofia. It had been quick and uneventful. Ten hours from arrival at the hospital to holding her in my arms. Mum had sat with me in the room for some of that time, and was the first family member to see the baby.

While the doctor was giving me my one, neat little stitch, my daughter lay on the left side of my chest and within a few seconds lifted her head, opened her eyes and stared at us with that cloudy newborn gaze. 'So, you're the parents, huh?'

People brought flowers and cupcakes. It's hard to remember a time when I felt happier.

There were no flowers and cupcakes where I was going now. The room was a mirror image of the one I'd stayed in when Sofia was born, but this section of the hospital was eerily quiet, devoid of the bustle and colour of the place where women give birth to live babies.

As I changed from my maternity dress into a hospital gown and got into the bed with its starched sheets and plastic mattress protector, the nurse explained the procedure.

She would insert a pessary full of hormones that would make my cervix dilate. She'd keep inserting them until the baby was born. There was no way of knowing how long that would take. I should settle in, enjoy the painkillers she was going to give me, eat whatever food I wanted and watch TV.

She inserted the pessary and said she'd be back to check on me soon. I remember her touching my shoulder as a gesture of care, the warm sensation lasting a few seconds.

It was going to be a potentially long wait. I tried to turn on the TV. Daniel looked at the laminated information sheet and discovered that you had to pay to use it. Not much money – a dollar an hour – but I'd never paid to watch episodes of *Law and Order* before.

I guess there's a first time for everything.

*

The Monday before Easter I found out our baby's heart had stopped at seventeen weeks. As my doctor searched across the surface of my protruding belly with his stethoscope, I knew something was wrong.

He sent me upstairs for a more thorough scan, and within seconds of seeing the image on the monitor above me I knew that the baby was dead. I whispered to myself 'no heartbeat, no heartbeat' as the nurse manoeuvred the buttons and knobs on the ultrasound machine.

Five weeks before, in that same room, the baby had waved its arms and legs at me, its heartbeat registering loud and clear. Now it looked like it was lying at the bottom of my womb, the way my daughter used to lie sleeping at the bottom of her baby-sling in the first months of her life.

The Monday before Easter was a perfect autumn day. I left the medical clinic in a half-stupor. I found my car parked around the corner and wondered whether to leave it there and walk home. Then I thought about the parking fine that would arrive in the mail in a few weeks' time, a nasty reminder of this moment. And so, I drove the few kilometres back to my house, trying to focus on driving, hoping not to compound this shocking loss with a car accident.

I walked into the house to find our babysitter Jocelyn folding laundry. I told her the news and she gave me a tearful hug. I went to find Sofia, who was sitting on the toilet, clad in her blue polka dot nightie. She was wearing her plastic sapphire drop earrings, a gift from a work trip I'd taken to Melbourne the week before.

I hated leaving her for work, and so I'd soften the blow for both of us by asking her what gift she wanted me to bring back. Her requests had been very specific on that occasion. Sapphire drop earrings. A book about a guinea pig. A giant chocolate freckle. It had taken me a few hours of searching the Melbourne shops, but I'd found all three items.

I perched on the side of the bath and cried in front of her. Crying was something she'd never really seen me do in earnest. The first three years of her life had been so happy, so relatively carefree. She stared into my face with her brown eyes, the only echo of me in her features, and said over and over, 'What's happened?' I told her the baby was gone and Mummy was sad. She replied with a simple, 'Oh.'

I had already started reading books to her about becoming a big sister, so she knew that a baby was on the way. Now things had changed. We put her Dora the Explorer undies back on and washed her hands. Her father came home soon after, and she knew for certain this was not like any other day.

I have always loved Easter. There is none of the stress and end-of-year fatigue of Christmas. When Easter comes, I am ready for less humidity and the change in the trees, the slow cooking, cinnamon and nutmeg, and the best possible chocolates I can afford.

I love the Easter story, too. It's the most moving story of the Bible. Christ is not a sermoniser or a man who can turn water into wine but a son and a friend. There are times when he is uncertain, scared, alone. He is betrayed and renounced by those he loves, those who said they loved him.

Sofia was born just before Easter, and the week the baby died, I was busy preparing for the party we would have in the park on Easter Saturday.

The next morning I woke up at 5 am, dressed in the dark and drove to Bondi Beach for a walk along the ocean front.

There is something immensely soothing about the sea's consistency. On your best day, on your worst day, it goes on, oblivious to you and your concerns. The tide goes in and out, the waves roll and crash.

It was cloudy and cool as I walked towards North Bondi, past the personal training groups, dedicated surfers and dog people.

After my walk and a coffee, I drove back home, we dropped Sofia at day care and headed to the hospital for my induction.

*

It took all day and most of the night, but finally the baby was born. At about one in the morning, I felt a sharp pain, a few contractions and then the baby slithered out. I told Daniel to get a nurse, but it was 1 am. It took time to find one.

I lay there on the bed, waiting, with the baby between my thighs. I could feel it lying there. I closed my eyes and remained as still as I possibly could. I would not look. I would not move.

I lay there for about five minutes and I felt every single second tick by.

The nurse came and took the baby's body and the stained sheets away. She had checked I didn't want to see it. I was adamant.

'We keep hand and foot prints on file just in case you change your mind,' she said gently.

Given we'd gone way past the twelve-week mark, we had already picked out a girl's name and a boy's name.

If I knew the sex, saw the baby, it would be worse than it already was. It would be the death of a desperately wanted child, a child who had a name, and not a shapeless horrible thing that had happened that I would find a way to recover from quickly.

I rolled over and fell asleep.

We left the hospital the next morning and walked home under cloudy skies.

The next day I had planned a long list of activities. Sofia was staying with my sister for a few days. We would use that time to redecorate her room. A new big-girl's bed and mattress and a doll's house as a gift for her third birthday. The birthday party would go ahead.

I cooked and cleaned and wielded an allen key and a glue gun, putting together a little miniature house complete with furniture and tiny wooden dolls, a family of four. We blew up balloons and put together party bags.

It was raining the day of the party, so we went ahead with the festivities but inside the house. Family and friends and ten kids with their parents crammed inside our little terrace. We had an Easter egg hunt in the bedrooms, and then party games and cake.

Looking back at the photos, I see I was still dressed in my maternity wear, hustling in the background, trying to avoid the camera. In the few photos that manage to capture my face, there is no sign of sadness. I'm smiling as Sofia blows out the candles and opens her presents. Or I am preoccupied with scooping up discarded wrapping paper and empty champagne glasses.

Underneath my maternity top, my breasts were leaking milk. Stupid body didn't get the memo.

I knew what I was doing, even then. Shielding Sofia from my sadness. I refused to let her birthday become about this little death.

But also, a subterranean, unacknowledged part of me must have been pushing to carry on as usual. No-one was going to step up and clear a space for me to grieve. Or perhaps it was all me. Perhaps I didn't even know how to ask for that space. Either way, I convinced myself this wasn't something worth grieving about.

*

For most of session two, I was sitting up cross-legged on the day bed, tissue in hand, while Julia and I talked.

We talked about the induction and everything that happened after. About all the hardship between that and the birth of the twins.

Julia spoke more this time, asking me a few questions. It felt less like the waking dream of session one and more like a long, free-flowing talk with a wise interlocutor.

'Who do you think taught you how to love?' she asked me.

'My nonna,' I replied immediately. 'She was the only person who loved me without hurting me.'

The only person whose love felt like a strong straight line, rather than a jagged edge.

I continued to talk about my sister. How I felt I hadn't loved and cared for and protected her enough when we were children.

'That's the biggest obstacle to me reaching any kind of self-compassion,' I told Julia. 'My guilt that I let her down.'

Julia turned her head to the side and let a few seconds tick by.

'What would happen if instead of seeing your sister as a helpless child to be protected, you saw her as a strong woman you could confide in?'

She was right of course. Emily was a grown woman. She was strong and clever. She had stepped up as an aunt the moment Sofia was born, when the twins were born and every step of the hard decade since then. She was my go-to person for support when my marriage was falling apart.

She wasn't asking for my protection. Not now, anyway. As a child she had, that time in the playground, as the first MDMA session had made me relive. 'Rebecca, I feel really sick.' I'd walked away, failed to see she needed help. But at least I'd felt terribly guilty when I realised what I'd done. That counted for something.

I resolved I would call her as soon as I got back to Sydney and tell her about the MDMA. Tell her how sorry I was for the past but that I needed to forgive myself for what I didn't do, and that she could help me. That I needed her help.

But for most of the time I sat with Julia, I spoke about the loneliness I felt. An immense loneliness that stretched from before I could remember, that I thought I'd left behind when Sofia was born. But it had returned with a vengeance by the time the twins were born.

The drug had me feeling something, a truth I couldn't acknowledge until that moment on Julia's day bed with the trees and the hills outside and the breeze coming through the sliding doors.

That with the birth of the twins I had what I had been longing for, worked for, struggled for and bled for. It had taken four years, but I had my children.

But I'd lost my mother along the way.

Miscarriage as metaphor

In the weeks after the induction, I put all my efforts into carrying on as normal. I took a break from work, but only so I could finish writing my memoir about my nonna, *The Italian Girl*. It seemed a fitting way to direct my energy and to subdue my disappointment and shock, to write this tribute to her. I walked a lot, kept taking all my prenatal vitamins.

My friends rallied. My sister too. The freezer was full of food. We ran out of flower vases. I leaned on a few friends who had been through the same experience.

I'm neither religious nor spiritual, but during this period a part of me wished I was. Where are the soothing rituals that mark the beginning and end of life when you are faithless? I guess you have to cobble them together on your own.

Of course, everyone – heathens and believers – struggles to know what to say when someone dies. And a stillbirth is a strange kind of death.

Those who kept it simple, said they were sorry and gave me a hug were the best. A few people said nothing, or pretended like nothing had happened. This silence hurt me the most, which was ironic given I was acting like nothing had happened.

I believed if I could just get pregnant again as soon as possible, everything would be okay.

Legally, if you lose a baby, even via an induction, before twenty weeks it's defined as a miscarriage rather than a stillbirth. I described to people what happened as a stillbirth because I'd actually given birth. Or I said I'd lost the baby, as if it was some kind of forgetfulness on my part.

The official paperwork described it as a miscarriage. Perhaps that's why the doctors I encountered were so blasé about the loss.

While the nurses who cared for me during the induction were kind and attentive, my obstetrician was a man in desperate need of some empathy training. He had called on the phone during the induction to check up on me.

'I don't want to know the sex of the baby,' I'd said to him. 'It's very important to me that I don't know.'

When I went back a few weeks after the induction for a check-up, I walked in and he was looking at my file. After a perfunctory hello and not even a 'How are you feeling?', he said, 'Well, you had a boy …'

'I told you I didn't want to know.' My voice was angry, but a few tears sprang up in my eyes despite my determination not to cry.

'It's better that you know,' he said with an insistent tone.

'Why is it better? Does the fact that it was a boy have anything to do with the baby's death?'

'No, we found no abnormalities. I just think in these cases it's better you know.'

There are a few times in your life when you say exactly the right thing at the right moment. This was one of those times.

'I believe on this issue I am the best judge of what's best for me,' I said to the doctor. 'Almost everything about this experience has been beyond my control, except how much information I wanted to have about the baby. I was very clear about not wanting to know the sex. You didn't listen.'

He muttered some quick apologies and looked at my file again.

Without making eye contact, he said, 'Like I said, the tests found no abnormalities. Miscarriages are common, especially in a geriatric pregnancy. I anticipate you will probably get pregnant again and you will carry a healthy baby to term, given your history.'

I stood up and left without saying thank you, paid his substantial fee grudgingly and made a mental note to find a new obstetrician as soon as possible.

This doctor was both right and wrong about what would happen next.

I got pregnant again three months after the induction. The first ultrasound at twelve weeks found no heartbeat. I miscarried a few days later, on the floor of the women's toilet next to the public hospital waiting room. I passed out on a gurney as I was being rushed into the emergency room, having lost a lot of blood. The last thing I remember seeing before the blackness was the concerned look on a nurse's face and the harsh white lights above her head.

I got pregnant again a few months later and again, the first ultrasound found no heartbeat. I miscarried in a toilet after a work meeting.

Recurrent miscarriage is something of a mystery to the medical profession. It's generally defined as three miscarriages, albeit increasingly two miscarriages are enough to be classified as recurrent miscarriage.

In some circumstances the causes of recurrent miscarriage can be easily identified and treated – the mother has lupus or blood clotting problems, uterine abnormalities or an 'incompetent cervix'. Diabetes, autoimmune disorders and polycystic ovarian syndrome can also cause miscarriages. Couples with inherited genetic disorders that cause chromosomal problems in the foetus are also in a high-risk category. Other miscarriages are due to chromosomal problems with the foetus itself, but thankfully, advances in genetic testing have made these cases easier to discover.

However, the majority of people who've suffered recurrent miscarriages, even after thorough testing, are left in the dark. In at least fifty per cent of cases, the causes are unknown.

Theories abound about the other causes of recurrent miscarriage, but at the time it was happening to me there was scant research. Could it be caused by a lack of vitamin C or D, problems with thyroid function, problems with progesterone levels? There is an emerging thesis that women with high levels of natural killer cells are more likely to experience recurrent miscarriage. That the cells, part of our immune response to fight viruses and tumours, attack the embryo instead, as if the embryo was a potential threat to the mother.

Even more tentative are theories that recurrent miscarriage can be caused by caffeine intake, stress and other so-called 'lifestyle factors'.

By the time I'd lost baby number two I'd read as much of the medical literature as I could find. I hated reading those studies about stress, lifestyle and caffeine intake. Coffee-fuelled, engaging work was my escape from thinking about getting pregnant, being pregnant, not being pregnant.

Quiet time with my only daughter wasn't the calming activity it usually was. I tried to hide my sadness from her. I couldn't even look at photos of her as a baby, it was so painful to remember the feeling of her at that age in my arms. She was getting bigger, harder to pick up, ready to be a big sister. I wanted her to be part of a clan. I wanted more children to help bring my family together, to fill it out and to raise it up and away from my own childhood. But fundamentally, I wanted more children because I loved being a mother and I felt if I didn't have more, it would be an aching regret for the rest of my life.

With each miscarriage I found it harder to talk about what I was going through. I didn't want anyone to pity me. I felt weakened, diminished by people's sympathy. And yet if they weren't sympathetic at all, I became furious. After miscarriage number two I started to withdraw from the topic with friends and family. There was nothing anyone could say that would make me feel better.

Only getting pregnant again would make me feel better.

Of course, I blamed myself.

*

In 1978, American writer Susan Sontag published an essay, 'Illness as Metaphor'. Sontag had aggressive breast cancer at forty-two and the essay was a response to her illness and the treatment, which included a radical mastectomy and chemotherapy. In the essay, she is critical of the language commonly used to describe physical illness, namely the way that it 'victim-blames'. As if the physical condition is a manifestation of the person's psychological problems, aberrant character traits and repressed passions.[20] I read Sontag's essay in university and absorbed all her reasoning. Until recently.

In his book *The Myth of Normal*, medical doctor and trauma specialist Gabor Maté respectfully challenges Sontag's thesis. He writes that while blaming people for their illness is unscientific, that doesn't necessarily mean there aren't discernible and provable connections between emotions, developmental histories and diseases. It's not a question of blame, he writes repeatedly, but a matter of understanding the bigger picture.

He points to the mounting evidence that women, especially self-denying women, are more likely to suffer from autoimmune conditions like lupus and Crohn's disease. Diseases associated with chronic inflammation in the body, which is itself associated with ongoing psychological stress.

Maté also devotes chapters in his book to the impacts of maternal stress on the foetus in utero. He points to the 'deluge of fresh information [underscoring] the crucial importance of women's physical environment, health, and emotional balance during pregnancy to the optimal development of the infant'.[21]

There is no evidence basis for what I am about to write, but I am going to write it anyway. I would never have let myself think it at the time, and would have railed against anyone even faintly suggesting anything like it.

But reading Maté, I started to wonder if maybe my poor, overwhelmed and unloved body didn't want me to have more children.

Perhaps, in some twisted way, it was trying to protect me. *Sorry, you need to look after yourself better before you add another person who needs looking after to the already long list.*

Or maybe it had become resentful, withholding. I had always had a hostile relationship with my body – that's an unremarkable comment by the way; it's so common for a woman to dislike her body. But more than the feeling of dissatisfaction with its size and shape, I derived intense happiness from punishing my body, from denying it food, comfort, rest. From looking at it in the mirror with disgust. Forcing it to throw up. Perhaps it was rebelling, like an angry adolescent.

After the third miscarriage there were no more natural pregnancies for months. It seemed my body had given up even trying and failing to bring a baby to term.

Then there were two rounds of IVF.

On the first round they had implanted the best embryo out of a small batch. When that didn't take, they threw in two poorer-grade embryos and told me not to get my hopes up.

They took.

At eight weeks I saw Baby A and Baby B swimming around in their own private gestational sacs. During every scan from that point on they were moving around, bouncing off each other, growing well, their tiny hearts ker-thumping.

That's what I meant when I wrote that I'd thrashed my way through blood, pain, needles and piles of money to get to that moment.

That's why every second of that last, long, hard pregnancy, I was terrified that the babies would die. That my tired, overwhelmed, unloved body would kill them. That's why the first MDMA session made me recall not just the joy of finally holding Stella in my arms, but also that fear.

The MDMA kept pulling me back to these moments for a reason.

The birth of Sofia and the hope of love, connection, a chance to heal my family.

The birth of the twins, longed for and beautiful, yes. But by then, the hopes were almost gone.

*

The second session with Julia was much harder for me. I felt more alone, more burdened by the legacy of my childhood and all the losses between that first easy birth and the last. Maybe it was because I was in an unfamiliar place. Safe, but still strange. Or perhaps this time, the MDMA was dragging me into colder, darker waters.

As I was packing up my bag to go back to my accommodation, Julia offered me a small jar of psilocybin capsules.

'They are going to help you over the next few days with integration. Take two in the morning before food.'

The beige capsules she handed me contained a combination of a range of powdered fungi. As with MDMA, I knew people who had taken mushrooms recreationally, but I'd never tried them myself. Like MDMA, psilocybin has been made legal in Australia to be prescribed in cases of severe depression and PTSD – another world first. When eaten, psilocybin is converted by the body into psilocin, which activates the same receptors in the brain that serotonin activates.[22] The psilocybin would help cushion that serotonin dip I'd experience in a few days. As well as to support the integration process in the coming weeks.

I took the bottle and put it in my cosmetic bag along with my lip balm and asthma inhaler, thinking how I would have to hide it well inside my luggage.

In the car, Julia and I talked about her impending departure. She was clearly going to miss her home, but some siren call she didn't reveal to me was chasing her away to other climes.

'Do you have any clients in the area?' I asked.

'Some. There are lots of people living here I'd like to work with and who would like to work with me, but they don't have enough security in their lives. Their living arrangements are still tenuous because of the floods.'

She didn't need to elaborate; I knew what she meant. The area we were driving through had recently been hit by one of Australia's biggest and most expensive natural disasters.[23] Between the end of February and the beginning of March 2022 the region experienced historically high rainfalls over seven local government areas. The town of Lismore was inundated. Rivers overran and the floods destroyed homes, community buildings, roads, businesses. A year on, locals were still reeling. It remained a massive task not just to work out how to rebuild, but to address the collective PTSD. The floods had come too soon after another catastrophic climate event, the 2020 Black Summer fires. Those megafires had burnt through parts of the Northern Rivers, along with 24.3 million hectares across the country.

The last book I had written had been about emotional responses to climate change. How we can effectively channel the fear, anger, hope and guilt we feel when we think about climate change into action. I'd had my own profound emotional response to climate change sitting on my couch one morning watching the School Strike 4 Climate protest in Sydney. Teenagers not much older than my eldest daughter demanding governments act to reduce the use of fossil fuels and protect nature. My reaction to the climate protests was a heady mixture of love and guilt. Here was my children's generation calling on their parents, calling on me, to act, to create a liveable world for them. The Black Summer fires soon after that turned me into a committed environmentalist, and now much of my work as a social researcher is spent helping governments, companies and not-for-profits with nature protection and energy transition campaigns.

In the research for my book, I came across a term coined by Professor Glenn Albrecht from Murdoch University in Western Australia: 'solastalgia'. It's a kind of environmental grief generated by losing important aspects of your home when it's been transformed by a climate event.[24] As Julia and I drove past the school and the houses I had walked past that morning, I thought about the people inside them and wondered how many were feeling this grief for lost places while still living in them. I'm not sure whether it was the lingering effects of the MDMA, but I could feel some of this grief riding on the back of the air that flowed through the car window.

I ate without appetite that evening, and afterwards sat on a beanbag by the pool weeping on the phone to my friend Sarah.

The aftermath of the first session had been a smooth experience in comparison to this. Even amid all the resurfaced memories of pain and loss, I managed to hold on to the warmth of the love my mother had showed me when I was sick in Oxford.

This time felt glum and cold in comparison. Like I was at the bottom of a deep, earthen well looking up at the sky. I lay in bed flicking through photos of the children on my phone, and finally fell asleep once the bush sounds overtook the noise of the other guests returning to their rooms.

I woke the next morning in much the same mood. The sun was already up and you could sense it would be another hot, humid day. I stepped out of the bedroom onto the porch for a stretch and to take in more of the view of the Pacific Ocean, hoping I might see one of the rare yellow-tailed black cockatoos that are supposed to live in the trees around the mountain.

Like I said before, I didn't grow up an outdoor child, but I turned myself into an outdoor person. Hiking in nature helped tame the whirligig for years, made me feel more together, as if my mind and body weren't at odds.

How many words have been written about the restorative power of natural places, of the symbiosis between humans and the natural world? About the fact that we forget that at our own peril. About how we are now in peril because so many of us live every day as if that isn't the stone cold, fundamental, God's honest truth.

Billions of words written and spoken and I am not sure I can improve on any of them. I can only write that I managed to lean on those trees and the sound of the ocean, the distant birdsong and the smell of the salt and eucalyptus oil in the air. It helped me summon the energy to shower, pack, eat and organise a taxi to get home.

At that moment, I felt disconnected from every human being, but I felt a deep and gratifying connection to that natural world.

If I'd been able to manage it without being seen by the other guests, I would have found a tree and hugged it.

Calling out for my mother

In the weeks after the second session, I thought a lot about birth and loss. About how I'd thought becoming a mother would bring me closer to Mum, when in fact the opposite had happened.

During my first pregnancy Mum seemed excited. She rang regularly to see how I was. When I went into labour she came to the hospital. She sat with me when Daniel went out for a walk or to get food, then she sat in the waiting room until Sofia was born.

She came to visit me in the hospital after the birth, while I was trying to get the hang of breastfeeding.

'You know I am going to be in and out of your house like

a blue-arsed fly for the next year,' she told me. I'd never heard that phrase come out of her mouth. Blue-arsed fly?

'Really? That's not necessary Mum, I can handle it.' I had no expectation of any help from my mother. All I wanted was time together.

'Once you are back at work, I'd like to look after her one day a week,' she said.

'That's a lot. I know you don't really like babies.'

'I don't like babies but I like this baby. She's my grandchild.'

My happiness at my mother's desire to be so involved in Sofia's care had an unstable quality to it. It felt like an outstretched hand that could be yanked back at any time. Still, I wanted to believe her. I imagined walks to the local cafe, just the three of us. I imagined filling an album with photos of Sofia's first year. Nonna and me. It could be my mother's Christmas gift. She was hard to buy for.

I returned to part-time work a few months after Sofia was born. I worked from home most mornings, and then Mum's day with Sofia would be my designated day in the office.

I had no illusions about being able to concentrate on work and look after a baby at the same time, so we interviewed for a nanny. The first person we met was Jocelyn. She was in her sixties, a grandmother and the most organised and energetic person I'd ever met. She'd been with a few families before us, long stints, which seemed like a good sign.

'I don't call myself a nanny. I'm a mother's help. I'm here to look after the baby but also you.'

'I'm fine, I don't need any help,' I said to her with a smile.

'Sure you do,' she smiled back. We hired her the next day.

Jocelyn would bustle in on time in the morning and, along with getting Sofia into an iron-clad routine of food, sleep, nappy changing, a walk and play, she would iron shirts, empty the dishwasher, hang out washing and later bring it inside, prepare rice pudding for Sofia and pick up any essential items we needed from the supermarket on her morning walk with the baby in her stroller.

When Sofia broke out in a terrible nappy rash, Jocelyn went to a compounding chemist to get a special barrier cream that sorted it within a few days.

I thought I had it made. Easy baby. Mother's help who was a godsend. And Mum bonding with Sofia once a week while I had time in the office.

'Why do you need a mother's help?' Mum asked when I told her about Jocelyn.

'I can't concentrate on work and the baby at the same time.'

'Well, I can help you.'

'It's fine, Mum, one day is more than enough.'

The first couple of weeks went smoothly. Mum picked up Sofia in the morning from my place and Daniel would pick her up on his way home from work. I didn't feel too guilty about the effort this required, as Mum had help from her partner and my sister. She wasn't doing this alone.

After a few weeks, I got a call from Mum.

'It's going to work better for me if you drop Sofia in the morning rather than me coming to you. There's a lot of traffic.' It meant an earlier start for us all, but fine. I was committed to making this routine work.

Six weeks into this arrangement I was at the office, cramming my lunchtime salad into my mouth as I checked my email when I got a call from Mum.

'When are you planning to get home?'

I was taken aback. It was a usual work day. Even leaving at five on the dot seemed like special treatment – most people were still at their desks at that time.

'Probably about five-thirty. Is everything alright?'

'Oh, it's all fine, everything's fine. I might just go back to your place now with Sofia and wait for you.'

I immediately told my boss I needed to leave.

By the time I got home, Mum was there sitting on the couch while Sofia was on the floor playing. Mum left quickly, saying she needed to pick up some shopping.

I felt like I'd done something wrong, but I was unsure what. It was that uneasy feeling I'd had my whole life, that I should be able to read her mind but couldn't. I knew if I asked her what was wrong, I'd be met with deflection.

Two days later, I got another phone call.

'I forgot to tell you I'm going away to Europe for a few months so I won't be available to look after Sofia.'

I was shocked, but not shocked. I'm not sure I said anything more than 'Where are you off to?' and 'Travel safe.' As soon as I was off the phone, I called Jocelyn to see if she could cover another morning and then rang around to the various childcare places where we were on the waitlist to see if we could start Sofia earlier.

Mum went on her holiday to Europe. When she returned, neither of us brought up regular babysitting again.

I would, if I was desperate, ask her for help.

One time, I had a work thing that couldn't be moved and that couldn't go ahead without me. Jocelyn couldn't cover, neither could Daniel, and my usual phone-a-friend options were exhausted.

I called Mum. Could she look after Sofia for a few hours? I could drop her off and pick her up.

Silence.

'I can on this occasion, yes. But I have noticed something, Rebecca.'

'What's that?'

'You only call me when you want help. It's like I only exist to help you.'

'That's not true, Mum. I call you all the time. You don't always call me back, or maybe you don't get the message.'

Mum didn't have a mobile phone, she never picked up the home phone and she rarely responded to email. If she wouldn't come to the phone, the only way to be sure she received a message was to drive over to her place and tell her face to face. Most messages were relayed through my sister and my mother's partner.

I hung up the phone feeling incredibly hurt and guilty. Was I just using Mum for what I needed? Perhaps in the busyness of juggling a baby, work, a marriage and everything else, I'd forgotten to make her feel loved.

I was determined to do more for her, to call her more and not to ask for help. I needed to prove that I didn't need her to help. I just wanted to have her in my life, for her to get to know my child.

I organised events, lunches, dinners, outings. I brought over gifts. Sometimes Mum would turn up, sometimes she'd cancel at the last minute, saying she was tired or felt unwell. I never confronted her about her behaviour. I just kept trying.

One night Sofia was unwell with one of those horrible chest infections. She was coughing and crying and couldn't settle. She would sleep soundly in a moving car, however, and so I drove around the neighbourhood streets in the wee hours of the morning, waiting for the grey light of dawn.

While driving along the main strip of shops near our house I saw a crappy-looking cafe with a heap of taxi drivers and police waiting for their breakfast rolls and cappuccinos. I stopped and pulled Sofia out of the car and onto my shoulder, moving carefully so she wouldn't wake up. I needed coffee, peanut butter toast, something to keep me going.

As I sat outside the cafe, Sofia grizzling in my arms, I spied the florist across the street unloading armfuls of tulips, roses and lilies from her little white van. I remembered the flower markets were open that day and I had the bright idea of going, grabbing all Mum's favourite flowers and dropping them over to her with some breakfast. If I was stuck driving around with a sick child, at least I could do something nice for someone.

An hour or so later I arrived on Mum's doorstep with a loaf of fresh bread and an armful of blue irises and yellow calla lilies. Sofia was asleep, strapped in her safety seat in the driveway with the door open.

I checked my watch – 8.15 am. Not too early.

I rang the doorbell and heard footsteps. The door opened, but only a few centimetres. Mum's partner peered out at me.

'Oh, hello Rebecca. Um, now's not a good time. Your mother isn't feeling well.'

'I'm sorry I didn't call. I just brought this stuff around for her. Can I bring it in? I'll put the flowers in a vase in her room and then I'll go.'

The door remained only slightly open.

'Um, well, she's not up for visitors.'

I was a visitor, yes, but I was also family. This was my family home. I stepped forward and pushed the door open. He let me through.

'I promise I'll just put the flowers in a vase and leave straight away.'

I dumped the bread in the kitchen and put the flowers in a tall vase with fresh water and some flower food.

I entered Mum's room and it was dark, full of the smell of the two brown Burmese that lay next to her on the bed.

Mum was half-sitting up, lying back on an abundance of pillows with the covers pulled up towards her shoulders.

She was staring at me with a kind of dark intensity I hadn't seen for years. As I put the vase on top of the TV cabinet opposite her, she didn't move or say anything.

'I'm sorry you aren't feeling well and I promise I won't stay. I've been driving around most of the night so Sofia can sleep, so I thought I might as well drop this stuff over from the flower markets.'

Silence.

'Mum, are you okay?'

A voice laden with contempt came out of this mask that was my mother's face somewhere in the half-darkness.

'Whenever you come to see me, you always bring nice things.'

'I do, yes.'

'You know what I think when you do that? I always think, I wonder what Rebecca wants from me now?'

I paused, trying to work out how to respond. I had clearly stumbled upon my mother in some kind of state of malevolence. Some kind of depressive fug that might be a one-off or might be recurring. No wonder her partner didn't want to let me in.

'I don't want anything, Mum. I just wanted to bring you flowers.'

She closed her eyes and turned over onto her side. One of the cats near her stirred a little and rearranged itself.

'I need to rest now, Rebecca.'

I slunk out of the room

*

Mum was one of the first people I called that Monday before Easter when the ultrasound revealed that the baby had died. She drove over with my sister and they dropped off food at the doorstep without knocking on the door. She checked up on me each day with a phone call.

But the first time I saw her in person was at Sofia's birthday party. Did we hug? Did she say she was sorry? Probably. I can't remember, but that doesn't mean it didn't happen. I was in some kind of daze that day, and for weeks after.

A few months later I got a call from my mother. I was driving two hours north of Sydney to speak at a conference.

'I wasn't even going to tell you this because I know how busy you are, but they found some pre-cancerous cells in my uterus. I need to have a full hysterectomy as soon as possible.'

'Mum, that's terrible. Will you need chemo or radio after?'

'The specialist doesn't think so. We got it early before it spread.'

'What can I do?'

'Nothing. It's fine. I'll be fine. Focus on your work and Sofia.'

I called my sister straight after and we talked. She sounded calm, repeating what Mum had said, that it was good they caught the cancer early.

'What do I do? Make meals, help in some way?' My sister and her partner lived on the top floor of our family home and Mum and her partner lived underneath. Emily said there were three adults around to assist; I wasn't needed.

Mum had the hysterectomy, the cancer was contained and there was no need for chemo or radio. I sent flowers after the operation. I called regularly.

Other than that, I did what I had been told to do. Nothing.

Mum never forgave me.

*

One great thing happened during that horrible year of cancer and miscarriages.

Daniel and I bought our first home. For the first time, we had a dining room big enough for a dining table that could fit twelve people. All the extended family, on both sides.

I remember seeing the table in the store. It was a French-style wooden kitchen table with turned legs. If it's possible to fall in love with a piece of furniture, I fell in love with this table. As we paid for it and organised for its delivery, I started to plan the menu for the Christmas lunch we would enjoy seated around it. All my nonna's special dishes, plus the traditional English fare that Daniel's family couldn't imagine Christmas without. Zuppa inglese and baked ham. Melanzane al forno and plum pudding.

I called Mum to tell her about the table.

'It's been a horrible year. The baby died and your health scare. I'm so stressed and tired. I'm really looking forward to having everyone around the table at Christmas.'

She agreed. I rang her often to ask how she was. I talked about Christmas, how imagining everyone around the table together was keeping me going.

In late November I was chatting to my father-in-law

over lunch. I started talking about Christmas, how much I was looking forward to it.

'Mum's had a terrible year, so I am going to cook all her mother's best dishes.'

He furrowed his brow a little in confusion.

'As I understand it, your mother is going to be away at Christmas. She is going on a cruise to New Zealand.'

'I don't think so. Maybe after Christmas. I talked to her the other day and she said nothing.'

'I think you'll find she's not going to be with you for Christmas.'

I did the thing I always did when things went wrong with my mother. I called my sister.

'Is Mum going on a cruise at Christmas?'

'Yes, she is.'

'Why didn't she tell me? I've been going on for months about how much I'm looking forward to Christmas and now she's not going to be there.'

'You need to talk to her,' was all Emily had to say.

Of course, I didn't. I was too hurt, bewildered, angry.

A few days before they were due to leave for their cruise, I dropped by the house with their Christmas gifts. Perhaps Emily had told them I was angry and hurt; Mum barely spoke to me, barely looked at me. I put the gifts in the hall, wished them bon voyage and left.

Mum didn't even get up from the couch to say goodbye, just shouted, 'See you when we get back,' down the hall.

Christmas was still fun. The table looked beautiful. We splurged on a real tree. I made the English menu, but not Nonna's dishes. That would have been too much to bear.

A couple of weeks passed and my resentment waned. Emily texted me that Mum had returned from New Zealand and I told her I'd come over with Sofia to say hello.

As I walked up the pathway towards the front door, I can honestly say I was excited to see Mum, and for Sofia to see her too. I'd made a cake, but maybe we'd go out for coffee? Just the three of us.

The door swung open before I could ring the bell and there was Mum, standing defiant in front of the door jamb.

'Well, have you recovered from your little tantrum about Christmas yet?'

Her voice was a snarl. Sofia was startled and burst into tears. I scooped her up.

'It wasn't a tantrum. I was hurt. You didn't tell me. I had to find out from Daniel's father.'

Mum slammed the door.

I walked quickly towards the car with Sofia still crying with shock in my arms. I sat in the back of the car holding her, trying not to cry, knowing that would make her more upset.

Breathe in, breathe out. What should I do? I couldn't walk away. I couldn't leave it like this.

I waited until Sofia was calm, then walked back to the house and rang the doorbell.

Her partner answered. He let us in and we went down to the lounge room where Mum was sitting on the couch, arms crossed, her face full of thunder.

'I deserved to go away if I wanted to. I was recovering from cancer. Not that you seemed to care at all.'

'I did care.'

'When your friend Meredith got cancer, you cooked for her and you cleaned her house. You didn't do anything for me.'

It was true. Fifteen years before, my friend Meredith was diagnosed with stage three cancer. She had an operation and a course of chemotherapy. Early on, she'd read some research saying that the more support from friends and family you get through treatment, the more likely the chance of a full recovery. She asked a select group of people to help out with chores while she was in and out of hospital. I felt chuffed to be asked. It felt like a gift to have something concrete to do rather than just worry about her and try to guess what might be useful. For four weeks I went over with takeaway, cleaned floors and wiped down bathrooms. I must have mentioned it to my mother.

'Mum, Meredith asked for help. You were adamant you didn't need any.'

'I shouldn't have to ask. You should just know what to do.'

I tried not to burst into tears of frustration. By then, Sofia was in the kitchen being entertained by my sister, who had made her way silently through the house a few minutes after I had sat down.

'Mum I'm sorry, but I have been so preoccupied and just, well, I lost a baby. I lost a baby and it's been so hard.'

Then I couldn't stop the tears. I sat there and sobbed. I hadn't really said those words out loud before, not to her or to anyone. Even saying it had been hard felt too much like an admission of weakness. Of vulnerability.

Mum sat, looking at me with a kind of dispassionate confusion, like I was a puzzle to be solved.

'Why do you want another child? You've already got a perfectly good child over there. I never wanted two children. In fact, I never really wanted any children at all.'

*

I always knew Mum found motherhood hard. It was, of course, forced upon her in a way. What working-class Italian girl growing up in the 1950s could have aspired to be anything other than a wife and mother?

I had always believed it was possible you could love your own children but also not want to be a mother. I always thought Mum's almost weekly revelations about how hard motherhood was, how ambivalent she felt about it, how much babies and children bored her, were the kind of honesty and candour that proved we were close.

She loved me enough to tell me these things.

Now I wasn't so sure these disclosures were a good thing.

After our fight about Christmas, I spoke to my mother less and less about trying to get pregnant, the miscarriages, the IVF.

I told her in a hurried phone call that I was pregnant with twins. She would call Daniel every few weeks to see how I was rather than call me. It was as if we couldn't speak directly to each other, only through other people.

A few weeks before I gave birth to the twins, she called me. 'I want you to know I've decided to go back to full-time work. The school really needs me.' She'd been retired for a year or so. She'd never actually worked full-time but I chose not to mention that to her. By then I knew a little about the game she was playing. The timing of her decision was not coincidental. She was trying to find a way to tell me, *Don't think you can rely on me now that you are about to become a mother again.*

She came to see the twins briefly in the hospital and afterwards, in their first year, only a handful of times at our house. Mostly I would drive them over to see her.

That's what I meant when I wrote that so much had changed between that first birth and the last one. That I finally had my family but I had lost my mother.

I couldn't see it at the time. I was so determined to create this new and improved, close and connected family that I didn't pause to ask myself if that was what my mother really wanted.

*

A few months after session two of the MDMA therapy, my daughter Sadie, at eight years old, became very sick.

It wasn't clear at the start of her illness, but she'd caught a virus, then a post-viral infection led to inflammation in the nodes of her stomach. It caused acute pain, and she was in and out of emergency for days as the medical staff tried to work out if it was a burst appendix.

No amount of over-the-counter medication or heat packs and warm baths could get the pain under control.

Finally, she was admitted to hospital. They put two cannulas into her slim little arms and started to pump different pain-relieving drugs into her, to no avail. Fentanyl and morphine didn't seem to work.

As the doctors were considering surgical options, Sadie's pain ramped up, and her spoken complaints escalated to screaming.

The nurses gave her ketamine, but all that did was make

her hallucinate and become even more distressed. She thought the medical staff had three eyes and were monsters trying to kill her. She thought she was dying.

'Mummy, I'm scared, make it stop. I feel like I am dying. Why does everyone have three eyes? Make it stop. Mummy, I love you. Make it stop.'

I found myself alone with my child in the middle of an almost surreal traumatic episode. I decided in that moment to handle it very differently than I might have if I hadn't been thinking so deeply about the connection between body and mind. How trauma is experienced through the body even when the memory of the trauma fades. And about the power of a mother's love when we are sick and scared.

I took off my shoes and lay down in the hospital bed. I put Sadie's body on top of mine, rested her torso on mine and opened my legs so hers could lie straight. I made myself into a kind of flesh La-Z-Boy for my daughter.

I lay with her like that on and off for four days while the medical staff took blood, did tests, poked and prodded her. I let her scratch at me and squeeze me and grab at my hair as the pain crackled through her body. I tried to remain calm, gently stroking her hairline during quieter moments. I tried to imagine all the pain and fear in her body crossing over to mine so I could absorb it, metabolise it, make it disappear. I did this for her but also for myself, to counter my own panic and distress.

In the first two days in the hospital, when we were still unsure what was truly wrong, while Sadie was sleeping, I would go and sit in the ward's playroom.

It was a square room made mostly of large windows, full of sad-looking, under-played-with toys. The children in this part of the hospital were all one step away from the emergency room – so, on the whole, too sick for Lego. I noticed the playroom was mostly where parents went, out of earshot of their children, to call relatives with updates.

I was sitting on a kid's plastic stool in the early hours of the morning on the second day, waiting for my friend Meredith, who was by then living in London, to call me back. I could hear the faint noises of the children in the other rooms. A toddler with tubes connected to his face and arm. Another child, bald and pale, all the signs of aggressive cancer. Another child who had been in a car accident. I heard their mewling and muffled cries, and they were all saying the same thing.

Mummy.

Even the toddlers who were pre-speech seemed to be crying out the same word. Mummy.

The common call of dying soldiers and sick children. And me.

I was exhausted. Hungry for a home-cooked meal. Wearing my sister's clothes that she'd brought for me to wear. The bottoms of my feet were black. I had taken my shoes off in the emergency ward and walked the halls of the public hospital barefoot for days without realising. I wasn't exactly sure where my shoes were.

I felt bereft. And in that moment, all I wanted was my mother. Just for her to be there. To tell me I was doing a good job and that Sadie would be alright. Even though other people – Daniel, my friends, my sister – had said that to me more than once, I knew nothing would have the power of those words spoken by her at this low, helpless moment.

That need for my mother was so primordial that it defied all logic.

My mother wasn't coming. Even if she had known her granddaughter was in the hospital, only ten minutes' drive from her house, she wouldn't have come. We hadn't spoken in over twelve months.

But this need for a mother's comfort never goes away. You might only ever experience that kind of care in a haphazard way in your lifetime, and yet the thirst for it remains with you forever.

Sadie's illness and the rough landing after session two had made me postpone my final session with Julia. I had always intended on doing a third session online with her mid-year but it wasn't until late August that I felt up to it.

As soon as Sadie was back at school and feeling better, I decided it was time to book that final session.

PART THREE

Dad, we hardly knew you

Despite the fact Dad made no appearance in my first MDMA session, I thought he might turn up in the second session.

But he didn't, and afterwards I started to think about why. It was possible that after all these years I had sufficiently dealt with his violence and cruelty. I'd been wise to make that definitive decision in the law school basement to give up on any hope of an honest relationship. I cared about him less than I did about my mother, so it followed that my subconscious fretted about him less. Mum was in my head and close to home physically, too, whereas Dad was not.

Ever since he'd left Australia for Cambridge, my father had played a walk-on part in my life. A minor speaking role at best.

In contrast to my relationship with my mother, there was a predictable rhythm to interactions with my father.

He sent cards with a cheque on birthdays and for Christmas. We'd get the occasional email from him, announcing the end of one marriage and the start of another, an adoption, another adoption, a pregnancy, then another divorce, another marriage, another pregnancy, and so on.

Even his rollercoaster personal life felt predictable after a while. I treated these emails like news reports from some intractable foreign conflict. Reasonable levels of concern and care without taking any of it personally.

He'd visit us when work brought him to Australia or when he was en route from Asia to America. One time he flew into Sydney for a few hours just for Father's Day brunch, between meetings in Malaysia and in Washington.

As the years progressed, with each fly-in, fly-out visit, he looked increasingly tired, worn down and old before his time. His weight fluctuated. He would fall asleep suddenly at lunchtime. He would drink a double espresso at dinner time. He would read a novel on a flight and then struggle to tell me what it was about the next day.

Then one year he emailed well in advance of a trip to Sydney asking if he could take Emily and me to dinner. He was explicit that it was a dinner for just the three of us. Usually, Daniel would be invited to these things, and he'd also extend the invitation to Mum. By then Mum and Dad were good at being sociable, even friendly.

Emily and I talked about the exclusivity of the invitation. Why was he seeking a private chat? It couldn't be because he was about to announce another divorce or marriage, or another child. We had found out about all of those events via email, sometimes after the event.

I'd booked a table for three at a Thai restaurant in the inner west, near where I was living and where Emily was now working at the University of Sydney. I knew the service would be swift and friendly, something very important to my father who could easily become insulted if waitstaff weren't attentive.

We met at the restaurant and Dad seemed his usual preoccupied and exhausted self. But he also seemed nervous, which was a twist.

After the fish cakes and a bottle of wine were delivered to the table, Dad mumbled his way towards what he'd come to Australia to say to us.

'I've been having some health problems. I've done a few rounds of tests and seen some specialists and I've been diagnosed with Parkinson's disease.'

He waved away our words of concern but he didn't shrug away my hand, which I placed on his arm.

'I'm on medication. I'm feeling good. Don't worry. It's not hereditary.'

That hadn't been my first worry, but it was good to know.

He changed the subject abruptly, and shut down any attempts we made to switch it back to his prognosis. Further questions about it were met with one- or two-word answers.

He drank almost the whole bottle of wine on his own, then finished the meal off with two espressos. He was in Sydney for two days before heading to Asia, then America, then Europe before the start of the academic term.

As soon as I got home, I called a friend of mine, a medical doctor, for her advice.

She told me she looked after a few Parkinson's patients, all of whom were doing well.

'Regular exercise, a good diet, plenty of sleep and rest. Limit caffeine and alcohol. Manage your stress. Most of my patients went into early retirement or cut down on work when they were diagnosed.'

I put down the phone knowing that, regardless of the wonders of modern medicine, if a lifestyle change was what would keep him alive, my father was already half-dead.

Dad was determined that his career goals would outrun his disease. He increased his efforts at work, if such a thing was possible. He travelled even more, determined to expedite his election to the International Court as Australia's representative.

Where before our relationship had a consistency – quick responses to any emails I sent, cards and cheques and a lunch or dinner once a year – his behaviour became erratic. He'd forget a significant birthday of mine (not even an email when I turned forty), then a few months later would buy Sofia an artist's print by Sidney Nolan, something that cost in excess of $15,000 at the time. She was four years old. The painting was the first and only gift he would ever buy her.

I'd try to take all this in my stride. Not because I'd reached some profound understanding of what happened to me growing up. Mostly I just didn't think about him, and mostly he left me alone so I didn't have to think about him. It was a kind of benevolent neglect, which I felt grateful for at some level. I was preoccupied with being a mother, a wife and my mother's daughter, and combining all that with my work.

The churning anger I'd felt towards him in my teens and twenties gave way to frustration in my thirties and then mild anxiety – for him and anyone in his orbit – from then on.

The frailer he became, the harder it was to sustain my adolescent rage.

One of the last times he visited Sydney I bought tickets for us to see *Aida* at the Opera House. He called me Becky, something he hadn't done since I was a kid. He kept smiling at me, laughing at my jokes, trying to put his arm around me. Strange behaviour for him.

At one point I turned to see him weeping during an aria, in the scene where Aida hides in the vault so she can die with her condemned father, Radamès.

'*La fatal pietra sovra me si chiuse.*'

The fatal stone now closes over me.

It was Mum who loved Italian opera, Dad who preferred the German greats, the Ring cycle. It was weird seeing him so moved by something he had once considered histrionic and too Italian for his tastes.

I looked at him in the glow of the stage lights as he lightly sobbed. He'd become soft. A shadow of the man who used to terrorise me as a child. I couldn't imagine him mustering the energy for one of his explosions.

And so, all of my previous anger, frustration and anxiety subsided, and morphed into something else.

Pity.

*

As I've mentioned before, growing up, I loved the movies. I watched all the classics on TV with Emily and my mother. Anything with Katharine Hepburn or Bette Davis in particular. I liked complex, difficult women in pants.

When I was old enough to take myself to the cinema, I saw everything I could, regardless of quality (I think I saw

Forrest Gump on the big screen three times). Posters of the movies I loved lined my bedroom walls as a teenager – *Jungle Fever, Dances with Wolves* (yes) and *Casablanca.*

At university, I did an honours degree in cinema so I could get credit for my obsession.

Cinema primed me for wildly unrealistic expectations of what might happen in my father's last few months of life, namely that he might ask me to visit him, to witness some kind of dying declaration at his bedside. A heartfelt request for forgiveness. Or a desperately needed affirmation that he had in fact been a good father.

Or he might bring himself to say 'I love you', something I can't recall him saying to me as a child or an adult.

For years, I worried about what I would say back to him. How much I would lie, because by then, the truth would be too late, too cruel. I wordsmithed it in my head countless times. I wanted to be kind, but could I stomach being dishonest?

'It's okay, Dad, you did your best. Thank you for everything, you should be so proud of what you've accomplished.' That's the best I could come up with.

The movies get a lot wrong. In my experience, people die as they have lived.

There was no urgent call to visit him on his deathbed.

There was, however, an email.

It was 2021 and my father was living in The Hague as a judge on the International Court, his lifelong goal achieved. It was the middle of the COVID-19 pandemic and his health seemed to be going downhill with each passing week. His wife sent a few photos of him and he was unrecognisable. He'd had numerous falls, hospitalisations and infections over the previous few years.

I was getting a steady stream of bad news about his condition from one of his brothers, my uncle Michael. After one hospitalisation, I asked to have a Zoom call with him. He was lying in a special bed on the ground floor of his house, his eyes half closed, his head pulled back, mouth gaping, shaking. It was a short call, and it was impossible to know if he even heard what I said, because he said nothing.

He hadn't asked to see me, but I fretted about going anyway. I had some money set aside for a mercy dash, but it was complicated. The news was full of reports of Australians finding it hard to return home if they left the country. Horror stories about quarantine. By this stage I was separated from Daniel and the custody arrangements were one week on, one week off. We were homeschooling. I couldn't just take off and work from a hotel room in Holland. I couldn't do the return trip in a week. If he was hospitalised, I might not be able to see him anyway given strict rules about visitors due to COVID.

One afternoon in late May, as I was preparing for the arrival of a dog trainer to help me tame our newly acquired cavoodle puppy, an email arrived from my father, which was a surprise. I hadn't heard from him in months. It was a long email, whole paragraphs rather than his usual few staccato sentences.

The email started with 'Dear Rebecca', then quickly launched into a series of paragraphs that laid out his estate planning and the complexities of a trust he had set up for his children. He promised that the trust would be resolved soon, which made me feel hugely relieved. Without that money, I had little hope of buying my own home in the local area post-divorce.

He wrote, 'I hope you will spend the money well for yourself and the children.'

Actually, I had planned to blow it all on hats, but okay.

Somewhere in all the legalese, there was a sentence that stood out: 'I'm proud of you.' He'd never written that or said it to me. To other people, yes, often – they reported back. But to me, no.

Then it ended: *Love Dad.*

That was it.

I called my sister. She'd received exactly the same email, except it started with the words 'Dear Emily'.

Later that day, while the dog trainer was showing me how to discourage Shadow from jumping up when I walked into the room, I got a call on my mobile.

It was my uncle Michael. Dad was dead.

'You were the love of his life,' Michael told me.

Funny how words you don't believe can still be meaningful.

I went back into the kitchen and told the dog trainer my dad had just died, and asked if we could finish the lesson another time. She scuttled off quickly.

I curled up on the couch with the dog and turned on the TV.

I never did learn how to keep Shadow from jumping for joy when I entered the room.

*

I have a lot of dear friends who had childhoods like mine. Different in the details, but the same in essence. Maybe we find each other. Then again, complex childhood trauma is pretty common.

A few of us like to talk about the TV show *Succession*, its deft portrait of family dysfunction. The explosive, ambitious father. The absent, acerbic mother. The children all angry, suspicious, vying for parental validation.

Spoiler alert. There is a scene in Season 4 as the Roy children gather to review the newspaper obituaries about their dead father and the daughter, Shiv, says to her brothers, 'Dad sounds amazing. I would have liked to have met Dad.'

Emily and I laugh about that. I think we said the same thing to each other a few days after Dad's death.

When Dad died, the obituaries poured in, published in major papers in Australia and around the world. Along with biographical details – born here, went to school there – and the list of his more impressive career achievements, some of these obituaries described him as a devoted father and grandfather. That made me snort. Even Dad wouldn't have described himself that way. Why do we feel this need to turn people into something they were not when they are dead? If ever there was a time for honesty, it's when the person who is gone can no longer be hurt by the truth.

Dad's career was stunning in its ferocious output, breadth and depth. The 21-year-old version of my father, starting his degree at the University of Adelaide with dreams of post-grad studies overseas, would have been awestruck if he'd been able to read these obituaries.

I'm sure he'd have been similarly shocked to know there would also be four wives and seven children, and that he would die a withered and collapsed version of his former self in his home in The Hague in his early seventies, before he could even finish his first term as a judge on the International Court of Justice.

While the obituaries left me cold, I loved the emails and messages from his former students around the world. Dad had been especially generous with his time with people from South America, Asia and Africa, as well as New Zealand and Australia. He'd remembered what it had been like to be an antipodean post-grad at Oxford. Nose pressed against the glass, looking in at the ruling class. A part of him liked to think of himself as an outsider even when he was wearing judge's robes.

'Doesn't that annoy you?' my friend Ilona asked me. 'That he made himself available for all these students and not for you?'

It didn't. It made me happy that, in the midst of his relentless pursuit of achievement, he'd actually been kind to real, live human beings. That his legacy amounted to more than just books and precedent. And children in therapy.

*

Dad was cremated and a ceremony was held in his honour at The Hague.

The world was still in the throes of COVID, so we didn't attend. Like good girls, Emily and I organised an event in his honour at the law school in Adelaide to recognise his career successes since he'd attended that institution as a young man. It was easy to celebrate Dad the Lawyer as opposed to Dad the Father. It felt like the right, final thing to do for him.

His family and colleagues gathered in the moot court near the portrait of him I had commissioned a few years earlier. The portrait shows him in a suit (of course) and a green tie, sitting in a chair, slightly bent over, looking straight ahead with his piercing blue eyes. Tsering, the young woman who painted it, magically captured a particular look I'd seen him give students a few times, those handful of times I'd seen him teach. The one when he was about to make their day by telling them they had answered a legal question to his satisfaction.

We also organised a memorial event in the Great Hall at the University of Sydney, but that was quickly cancelled as the next COVID wave broke over the country.

Almost a year after his death, the memorial went ahead. Former students and colleagues would speak. A few of his favourite pieces of music would be played.

I was slated to speak, too. Just as I had fretted about what to say to him on his deathbed, I also worried about what words to use here.

Could I find a way to speak with honesty about the parts of my father that weren't associated with his career, his crushing ambition?

I wrote something the day after his death, and emailed it to my sister for her approval. 'It's perfect,' she wrote back.

I practised it a few times leading up to the memorial. I was nervous. I'd seen the RSVP list. My mother would be in the audience. I hadn't seen or spoken to her in months. I'd have to find a spot to look at while I was delivering the speech, somewhere I couldn't lock eyes with her. Not much manages to knock me off course when I'm speaking in public, but seeing her face, stripped of emotion or full of anger or sneering contempt, that would do it.

I woke up on the day to find Stella had crawled into bed with me. She had a fever, and I could see that her throat was sore and inflamed. Sadie complained of similar symptoms but showed no signs of illness. More like a severe case of FOMO, brought on by thoughts of her twin enjoying a day in Mum's bed with the iPad.

I decided to stay home. Dad's widow would speak about Dad, the man. That would suffice.

For what it's worth, here's what I was going to say …

It's with great sadness and pride that I stand up today to say a few words about my father.

Not as an academic, lawyer or judge. Others have spoken eloquently today about him in that context.

But Dad as a person.

My father loved cheese and red wine. He loved theatre, literature and history. He loved art from all periods and all cultures. He introduced his children to First Nations painting, African masks, modern art from Europe and English antiques.

He loved classical music. As children we would drive around with him in his yellow Volvo and he would have the music up loud, steering with one hand and conducting an imaginary orchestra with the other, vigorously waving two fingers in the air. On more than one occasion, stopped at the traffic lights, a pedestrian passing in front of him thought he was making an obscene gesture. The pedestrian would often return the favour but Dad wouldn't notice, transported as he was by the sounds of Mahler, Dvořák and Sibelius.

He had a silly sense of humour. He loved Monty Python and The Goon Show. *Each night in our house by the sea in Adelaide he would read my sister and I poems from Ogden Nash and AA Milne and he would laugh more than we would.*

He was the Australian cricket team's greatest fan whilst also being Australia's worst cricketer. I recall a hot day in Centennial Park and an academics versus students cricket match in which Dad spent two hours at the crease and got about eleven runs. I remember as well the looks of unrestrained delight on the faces of the students that this man they admired so much was, in fact, bad at something.

He tried to instil in his children a love of learning, a respect for intellect and a belief in the critical role of universities in public life. And, of course, the pursuit of excellence. He had high standards for himself and for us. He was not easy to impress. If you came home with 98 per cent in an exam, he'd show high levels of curiosity about the 2 per cent you screwed up. He always wanted you to get 100 per cent.

I can't speak to the substance of his legacy to international law, as I have said.

But I can speak about what he taught me about being both a proud Australian and a good international citizen.

He saw the two as connected. He loved this country and believed we should play a leadership role as an independent-minded, middle power on the international stage. That it was in our national interest to be an enthusiastic and constructive participant in the organisations he dedicated so much of his intellectual energy and time to: the United Nations, UNESCO, the International Court of Justice and the International Criminal Court.

So he was a patriot and an internationalist.

I never saw him angrier or more frustrated than when Australia lost at the cricket to England and when Australia followed England and the United States into the war in Iraq in violation of international law.

He wanted Australia to be big hearted and high minded. He always wanted Australia to strive for excellence, to achieve 100 per cent.

My father would try every year to return to Australia to see family and friends.

Illness and COVID meant he wasn't able to make the trip for the last two years of his life. COVID meant we couldn't get to him in the last few months of his life.

I think about what I would have said to him if I could have seen him.

I think I would have held his hand and said, congratulations Dad, well done, you got 100 per cent.

You did all that you set out to achieve.

And from this day on, for generations to come, every international lawyer, every international law student, will owe you a debt of gratitude for your hard work and your brilliance.

*

The memorial was streamed live on Zoom so people around Australia and the world, his many colleagues, students and admirers, could watch. Stella and Sadie and I squeezed into my bed to listen.

'They are saying such nice things about your dad,' Sadie said at one stage. 'Are they true?'

My children had only met my father a handful of times. He was never 'Grandpa' to them, only 'your dad'. I'd been as honest as was age-appropriate about our relationship. The beautiful things people were saying about him on Zoom seemed at odds with my portrait of him.

'They are true. He did good things. Some people loved him a lot. But he also did bad things. He didn't mean to hurt people. But he did anyway.'

I don't remember much about the service except one telling anecdote from his widow's eulogy.

She said Dad had advised her that, once he was gone, she should channel all her sadness and grief and despair into work.

'Work hard. It will help you forget the pain.'

Session three

My final MDMA session would be at home and online.

Julia had no planned return date to Australia. In the weeks after session two, she was travelling through various parts of southern Europe and Africa. In the background of my video calls with her, I got a peep into the life of a highly experienced, globe-trotting psychedelic healer.

For a microsecond, I imagined a life like that for myself, one without children or dogs, where I traipsed from country to country with a backpack and a confidential client list. Would I hide the medicine in a bag in some orifice to take across borders, or would I have a dealer in every port?

I couldn't wait for Julia to return to Australia and at that point, I didn't trust anyone else to help me. My MDMA experiences were tied up with her, and I wondered if the same drug with a different person would be less effective. We'd met twice face to face and developed enough of a rapport to make a virtual session work. I knew what to expect from the process. And I would be at home, safe and secure in familiar surroundings.

They say 'psychedelic therapy is only as safe as the therapist providing it'.[25] I'd come to associate all of the MDMA's positive impacts with Julia's energy and guidance. She was an unexpected complement to my work with my therapist, Karen. They were very different characters, but they ended up collaborating in a way, talking to each other through me. I'd tell Karen Julia's questions and observations, and I'd talk to Julia about what insights ten years of therapy with Karen had revealed.

The clinical trials on MDMA involved three discrete MDMA sessions, and from the beginning Julia had suggested a course of three, with breaks for recovery and integration in between.

To me, there is something about three.

Something that feels natural, inevitable, even poetic.

Newton's Three Laws. The Holy Trinity. The Bee Gees.

Three children born healthy. Three babies that never were.

The third and final session required a different kind of lead-up from the others. More planning on Julia's end, given that she wouldn't physically be there and I would need to prepare all the kit to make the session happen.

She sent me her eight-hour curated soundtrack so I could play it while she guided me via the secure Signal link.

I wondered how she'd get the MDMA to me. Easy. Two days after we agreed on the date for this final session, a box arrived containing a heavy, opaque glass jar with a black plastic lid. Inside the jar were two little capsules in tiny plastic bags labelled 1 and 2.

We had to start late in the day, as Julia was working in a different time zone. She wanted to ensure there was someone in the house supporting me, so I organised for one friend to take the first shift and another to take the second. They'd sit downstairs and watch Netflix while I sat upstairs, crying and tripping in the new pyjamas I'd bought for the occasion. Julia had their contacts on Signal too, so she could communicate with them if necessary.

It was in the middle of winter in Australia, so I had an oil heater in the room and more blankets close to hand. I had water too, and my mobile phone in case our connection via the laptop became unstable.

I was anxious in a different way than I had been before the previous sessions. I was still fresh from Sadie's pain crisis. The memories of her screaming for me in panic and fear, the days of uncertainty. By the time I was planning this last session she had improved, thanks to weekly sessions of therapy and visits to a paediatrician. I'd bought her a therapy dog, a black fluffball she called Nova. I had hoped all the drugs would mean the memories of her hospital stay were hazy, but she remembered every detail. We spoke about it often. I wondered if the MDMA would make me relive those horrible days in hospital, and the weeks after. I wasn't ready for that.

Once my friend Ilona arrived and set herself up downstairs, I went upstairs to my bedroom, got into bed and connected with Julia via the laptop.

She was somewhere in South Africa, the same kind of light flowing into the Zoom frame that I'd seen when we first connected.

There was no need for much small talk. We got straight to it.

I took capsule number one and lay back, believing now that the medicine would work and trusting that wherever it took me would be where I needed to go.

*

When I was writing my memoir about my nonna, *The Italian Girl*, I was constrained by having very few primary sources to rely on. No journals, letters, notebooks or home movies. Only a few photos and stories, passed down by both reliable and unreliable narrators. My relatives were too busy working to write journals, and their literacy skills were minimal.

Even if they'd had the time to write about their lives, I expect the papers would have disintegrated in the humidity of the far north. What the insects didn't consume, the mould would have eventually destroyed.

There were history books to help me, as well as a useful bundle of documents to be found in the National Archives. All the internment files of the men in my family, my great-grandfathers on both sides, and my own nonno Oreste, my mother's father.

As soon as war was declared, the Australian government started to intern Italians living in Australia, along with Germans and Japanese-born residents. But it wasn't until around the fall of Singapore that they started to intern people in large numbers, especially in north Queensland.

My nonna's father, Luigi – despite being a naturalised British citizen and a long-time resident of Australia – was interned in the South Australian bush, along with almost all of my male relatives, including Oreste.

When I was writing the book, no family member who witnessed my great grandfather Luigi's arrest was alive. There was no-one to tell me the story of how it went down. Of course, Mum had said her family didn't speak much about those terrible, uncertain years. The war ended, the men returned to the farms, kept working and kept largely silent about what had happened.

I was lucky that the police reports of Luigi's arrest were in the National Archives, publicly available and digitised.

When the war started, legislation was passed restricting the freedoms of enemy aliens.[26] Among many stipulations about where they could go and what they could own, an enemy alien was not allowed to possess a camera. It was thought that cameras could be used by fifth columnists to spy on homeland war efforts.

The police reports of my great-grandfather's arrest show he was taken from the family farm in South Johnstone, where he lived with his wife, Marietta, and my nonna, on 14 October 1941. As part of the arrest, they thoroughly searched the property. They found four cameras, three pairs of binoculars and a radio set, all prohibited for enemy aliens to own without written permission from the police.

The police reports show that while they were tearing apart my nonna's family home, her mother, Marietta, was in the garden trying to bury one of the cameras. A police sergeant at the scene wrote in the official report of the arrest:

> *While we were searching the premises, I noticed Mrs. Ballini trying to plant some rubbish down the back yard. I informed Det. Hird, who had a look and found 1 camera and a pair of binoculars. Mrs. Ballini was trying to hide the articles, so that we would not be able to find them. This is an example of how cunning these people are.*

The report on the search concluded that while there was 'no evidence available to prove [Luigi] Ballini is engaged in any subversive activities ... he would aid the enemy should he be given an opportunity'.[27] Luigi was loaded into the police van after they confiscated all the contraband and all his financial papers. My nonna wouldn't see her father again for another two years.

I told Mum about the story, about how her grandmother tried to hide a camera in the garden and was caught by the police who'd been sent to the farm to arrest her grandfather.

'That was Nonna's camera,' Mum said. 'Your nonna. She loved taking photos. She would develop her own photos on the farm. She used to tell me how much she enjoyed watching the images magically appear before her, picking just the right moment to pull them out of the solution so they wouldn't be under or over exposed.'

On the rare occasions when family members would discuss what happened during the war, Nonna used to always say, 'They took my camera.'

'Nonna was dying to give me a camera for my twenty-first birthday,' Mum said, 'but I had no interest in photography.'

I wrote about this incident in *The Italian Girl* and had all but forgotten about it since. Until the MDMA reminded me.

Fifteen or so minutes after taking the first dose, I was there on the farm in South Johnstone, standing in the dirt.

Watching my great-grandmother Marietta try to bury the camera in her sprawling vegetable patch full of herbs, zucchini and beans.

My nonna Teresa watching with trepidation from the wide wooden porch.

It was as if I could read my nonna's thoughts.

I don't feel safe here. In this country that doesn't want me. Anything I love can be taken away from me at any time.

And I felt her despair, the sense of injustice but also the futility of that, knowing that this was how the world worked for a poor, uneducated Italian woman on a cane farm in the middle of northern Queensland during the war.

I felt stuck in that scene. Frozen. Not like the fluid movement of my other MDMA-induced memories. Like I'd been cut and pasted into one of the small, square, black-and-white family photos I kept in tissue paper in a box in the cupboard.

I'm not safe here. Had Nonna ever felt safe again? Is it possible to restore a sense of safety once you've become an 'enemy alien'? Are you ever anything else?

Then I was out of the photo frame, no longer standing on the dirt of the South Johnstone farm but in my mother's bedroom.

In the period between when Dad left when I was fourteen and when I first left home at twenty-one, my mother and I would fight a lot. Sometimes about the expected things parents and teenagers fight about. I wanted freedom to go to parties and be with my friends.

But I was also angry at her. For not stopping my father from hurting me.

The MDMA led me back there, back in the middle of one of those fights about something I can't recall. I was yelling. So was Mum.

She was standing close to her bed and I was standing a half a metre away from her. My frustration reached its zenith and I grabbed the telephone from her bedside table, lifted it up to chest height and hurled it onto the carpeted floor.

The plastic mouthpiece, attached to the body of the phone by a long, curly cord, bounced and hit my mother on her elbow.

She yelped and I ran away in shock. I'd never touched my mother in anger before and now I had thrown something, and it had hit her.

I ran out the door, down the street and towards the bus stop. I sat on an empty bench and thought about where I could go. I was walking distance from my friend Deanne's house, but I was worried about what her parents might say if I turned up there unannounced.

I was at a loss about what to do. In the past when Mum and I had fought, I'd taken the bus up the road to my school.

There were no bolted doors preventing me from reaching my French classroom, which looked out onto the quadrangle. Sometimes the door would be unlocked and so I would lie on the ground, underneath the table where I usually sat conjugating verbs during the day.

Je fâche. Tu fâches. Nous fâchons.

I would lie there, out of the cold, and try to sleep. I'd only last a few hours before heading home again. The last time I'd tried to break into the French room it had been locked, so my only option had been to go home.

But on this night, in my haste to get away, I'd forgotten to bring any money for the bus. I walked up and down the main strip of shops in my neighbourhood. It began to get dark. I'd been away for hours by the time I walked back into the house. My mother was lying on her bed, arms crossed with that familiar frozen face.

Before I could say a word of apology or renewed anger, she said,

'I called the police.'

There was a split second between that sentence and the next one. Less than a breath or a beat of the heart.

She went on.

'I asked them what I would need to do to get a restraining order given your violence towards me. I have all the details I need. If I go ahead, you won't be able to live here anymore.

What's more, you'll have a criminal record and there will be no point going to law school because you won't be able to practise law.'

This was not a resurfaced memory. It was a pressing one. I'd thought about it a lot over the years, told it to friends, recounted it to my therapist more than once.

What I had forgotten, what the MDMA made me remember, was that in that split second, that breath, that beat of the heart between 'I called the police' and 'restraining order', I thought that she had called the police because she was worried about where I was.

I remembered the tiny lift in my chest.

I ran out and she called the police because she was worried about me.

Then the crashing down. Nup, that's not why.

I'm not safe here. In this house where people don't want me. The roof above my head, the floor beneath my feet can be taken away from me at any time.

Then I'm still in my mother's room but have jumped back in time. I'm not an angry seventeen-year-old anymore; I'm fourteen. Angry at my father, yes, but still idolising my mother.

Mum is in the middle of the bed, under the covers. It's broad daylight but the blinds are drawn and the room is dark. Emily sits on one side of her, I'm on the other.

We are jammed in close together, not because there's not enough room on her king-sized bed but because we are watching her closely. Trying to hold her up.

Mum has that blank, thousand-yard stare I'm so familiar with. She's motionless, deeply sad. Not crying, but she doesn't need to cry for me to know the extent of her desolation.

A few hours before this, the three of us had gone to the local ATM to see if the first of Dad's child support payments had arrived. The financial agreement had just been signed. Mum kept the house, the investment properties and had full custody of us. He would cover the costs of her medical insurance for life. He was supposed to pay a few hundred dollars a fortnight for our maintenance.

I remember the anxiety as we stood beside Mum while she punched in her PIN. The balance flashed onto the screen. The money hadn't arrived.

'It's not there,' she said in a flat tone. After this trip to the ATM, we were supposed to go to our usual cafe for morning tea, but instead we went home.

Mum crawled into bed and we followed.

Her silence was worse than anything, worse than angry words or tears.

Then she spoke into the dark space between my sister and me, without looking at either of us, although I sometimes wonder whether, in fact, she tilted her head slightly in my direction.

'You have sucked the life out of me.'

*

I'd been lying back on the pillows up until this point in the session. When I sat up, I realised the music had glitched and stopped at some stage, so the room was quiet. I checked the time on the laptop. Over two hours had passed.

Julia was still in the Zoom frame, eyes on me. The sunshine had moved to high above her head, bathing her in light.

'I get it,' I said to Julia. 'I get it. I get her now. I get why. My mother didn't feel safe around me. I never made her feel safe.'

Like I said, Mum was born into a hostile environment – the heat and the crocodiles, the nuns and the town racists, the hard labour and the threat of poverty without it. Born into a family of enemy aliens. Her first memory was of pain and blood inflicted by her father.

Growing up a working-class Italian woman in the 1950s and 1960s, assuming (often correctly) that the people she met thought she was stupid. No greater aspirations than marriage and children.

Marriage was all she had dreaded it would be. Shouldered with all the domestic and caring work. Full of loneliness, then betrayal and humiliation. Caught in a cycle of violence, if not directed at her, at her children.

Then left to raise these two children on her own, one of them capable of matching her in anger and resentment towards her parents. Motherhood had always been hard, but now it was even harder.

No-one really taught her how to love, how to give it or receive it with an open, optimistic heart. She regarded the whole world through a lens of suspicion. The whole world included me.

'Everything I was trying to do, all my efforts, the gifts and dinners and parties thrown for her, she couldn't see them for what they were,' I told Julia. 'Acts of love. I wanted us to be a family. I wanted us to be close. It seemed she could only see them as manoeuvres in a game.'

I pulled another blanket over me, took the second dose and Julia and I talked until late into the evening.

When it was all over, I thanked her profusely, trying and failing to find the right words to express the extent of my gratitude. Thanks to the wisdom of the medicine and her stewardship over the process, I'd gained a level of insight and acceptance about what had happened to me that I couldn't have imagined possible in the short time since we'd met.

'You're welcome,' she said simply.

I woke the next morning with none of the deep depression I had felt in the aftermath of the second session, nor the peace and quiet I'd felt after the first.

The whirligig was turning, but softly, slowly. In a way I could live with.

I walked the dogs down the street and towards the pathway along the bay, thinking about what was next. More therapy with Karen. More rest. More walking and time with friends. And more time. I'd get there.

There was something about the magic of three. The third session had helped me quash a nagging doubt that had surfaced on occasion. That I could have done more. Could have had one more conversation with my mother in which I begged her again for more honesty and trust, for better communication. Made a greater effort in terms of calling her, visiting her with food, buying her gifts. I could have found a way to read her mind, read between the lines, anticipate what she needed. Not reacted when she hurt me. Tried harder to make her understand me, who I really was.

It wouldn't have mattered. I tried for fifty years. It was time to stop trying.

Then I recalled something Mum had said once at the tail end of a huge family blow-up only a few years previously.

She'd brought up my behaviour after Dad left yet again, how hard our fighting had made an already difficult situation for her.

She said, 'I couldn't understand why you wouldn't just leave me alone.'

Safe as houses

A few weeks before Mother's Day in 2022, I stopped talking to my mother.

I have been working my way up to telling you this story, trying to find the right words to explain it, because even now when I write those words or say them out loud, it feels like they can't be true. Like I've stepped into a parallel universe.

I don't see or speak to my mother, who lives only a thirty-minute drive from my home.

If you believe in the multiverse, there are hundreds of versions of me out there, still calling her up when I am upset, seeing her, buying her gifts, cooking for her, crying over her, raging against her behind closed doors or to her face.

I imagine there might be a dimension where at a young age I arrived at a deeper understanding about her. Who she is, rather than who I wanted her to be. Where I understand and accept the limits of her capacity to love. Where I am still in contact with her, but in ways where I protect my sanity and retain my equilibrium. A universe where MDMA is legal and there are thousands of Julias in clinics all over the world helping and healing people.

In this reality, however, there is no contact. I used to say to people that I don't talk to my mother anymore. That I cut her off. But in reality, it was mutual. So now I say, we are not in contact.

Looking back, I can see that the end of my marriage helped bring about the end of things with Mum. Because that was when, for the first time in a long time, I asked her for help.

It was during COVID when Daniel and I separated, and we'd made the decision to keep the kids living in the family home for at least six months. Daniel and I would cycle in and out. During off-weeks, when I didn't have custody, I needed somewhere to stay.

Mum had a spare room, but I didn't ask to move in and she didn't offer. She was in remission from stage three breast cancer at that point and she was part of a clinical trial; as I understood it, the drugs that were part of the trial lowered her immune system. If she caught COVID, especially with her history of asthma and chest infections, it could be fatal. I couldn't come and go from the house and risk exposing her.

When I called Mum to tell her my marriage was over, the first words out of her mouth were:

'Whatever you do, don't sell the house.'

'Mum, that's just not possible. We have a mortgage and I can't afford to buy Daniel out of his share. I'll have to sell it eventually.'

What to do with the house was the last thing on my mind at that moment. Easing the children into the new regime was my biggest priority.

I did need a place to live in during non-custody week, though. Mum offered to find me a rental apartment and to cover the expense. I was surprised and grateful, and I accepted, without demurring and without much anxiety. These were extraordinary circumstances, a divorce during the pandemic. She genuinely sounded worried about me.

In the following days Mum kept sending me links to various apartments near the suburb where we lived. I saw one that looked good and emailed back to say, 'This one please,' and could she contact the agent for me? A few days passed and I called her.

'Did you manage to contact the agent about the apartment?' At that point in the pandemic, open inspections had stopped. If you wanted to rent an apartment you needed to contact the agent for a one-off visit.

'No.' She sounded pissed off.

'I'm sorry, we must have got our wires crossed, I've been so distracted. I thought we were going to go with that place?' A quick search on the web while we were talking showed it had already been snapped up.

'Perhaps you should find a place you like, Rebecca, and then I'll cover the costs as I promised.'

She sounded annoyed, but I pushed any questions about why to the side and started searching for places at the price point of the ones she'd originally sent me. I found one and emailed her the listing.

She shot an email back.

'That's too expensive.'

Eventually I found a studio apartment for $400 a week. It was basically two rooms and a bathroom, but it was clean and, more importantly, it included a fridge. I had no whitegoods and very little furniture to start this new, separate life.

I forwarded the link to Mum saying I'd found a place for $400 a week and gave her the date when the first payment was due.

The rental date came and went. No money from Mum. I thought about not raising it with her. Money was a constant worry now, but I could afford to cover the rent on my own if need be. I gave it one last go. I called her.

'Has the transfer been organised?'

'I don't know,' she said. She sounded so annoyed. 'I'll check.'

The next day the money arrived. Three hundred dollars. I wasn't sure if the reduced amount was deliberate or not, but I just took it in relief. It would help. At that moment in my life, every cent helped. I had to start again from the same financial position I'd been in when I was last single, over fifteen years earlier.

I thought back about the wisdom of taking up her offer to help. Was I dumb? Should I have turned her down? I guess I was anxious, desperately worried about the financial uncertainty of the next few years. And I assumed she could afford it.

See, by this point in her life, Mum was a multi-millionaire property owner.

When Dad left, Mum worked hard and fast to make sure she was financially secure. In addition to owning the family home and an investment property, she inherited property from her parents when they died. Nonna and Nonno arrived in this country poor, but over the years they did what wogs often did. Worked hard, bought land, bought houses that needed some TLC, renovated them, and then rented them to people who couldn't afford to own their own home.

But that seemed like it wasn't enough for Mum. I guess she wanted to make sure she never had to worry about the account balance on the ATM screen ever again. In the years after Dad left, she hustled like I'd never seen her hustle before or since. She was smart and motivated and managed, using the equity in the properties she already had, to buy four large houses in suburbs close to the Sydney CBD. It was the 1980s and gentrification hadn't yet hit these suburbs with their dilapidated terraces and public housing blocks.

In the years that followed, more properties were bought, a few others sold. I was never really sure or, to be honest, particularly interested. But I felt proud, and pleased for her. In the wake of a terrible marriage that could have left her, a Catholic school teacher working part-time, facing financial stress, she had become rich.

Mum would often say to me, 'I stayed in the marriage for you and Emily. I didn't want to lose all the property.' Or, 'I wanted to give you a house when you moved out so you'd always have a roof over your head.' Other times, 'You will be a wealthy woman when I die thanks to me.'

'You'll never have to worry about having a roof over your head' was the statement that confused me the most. She'd say it and I'd think about all the times I'd run away from home, the times I'd walked the streets not wanting to go back home, but at a loss as to where else I could go.

She had no idea that I'd worried about that roof over my head all my life.

Once I reached my early thirties, she did in fact help me with that roof, like she'd said she would. In the first years of our relationship, Daniel and I lived in an apartment she owned, paying about three-quarters of the rent she could have got on the open market. When Sofia was born, we renovated and lived in another house she owned in the inner-west suburb of Glebe. We also paid rent there, and when we finally bought our own home, she reimbursed us for the money we'd spent on the renovation.

We were grateful, and knew how lucky we were to have her support. Even back then, the Sydney rental market was soul-destroying. Weekly rent in our area was equivalent to having to service a half a million-dollar mortgage. There were long lines at open inspections and rental auctions, where people just kept offering more and more rent to secure a property.

In that horrible year of the stillbirth and cancer, the bright spot came when I sold some shares in Dad's family company and, with money from Daniel and money from Mum, we bought a lovely three-bedroom home near Sofia's primary school, close to our friends and the life we had created in the inner west.

I loved that house. I remember unpacking the kitchen and thinking to myself, *This is it. I've arrived. And I will never have to ask my parents for anything ever again.*

If only life turned out just like you wanted it to.

If you are Australian and reading this, you'll know something about the property market in Sydney. If you aren't, you might be in for a shock. Sydney regularly ranks as one of the most expensive property markets in the world, up there with London, Tokyo and New York. The median house price in Sydney is $1.6 million. In my neighbourhood, the median is above $2 million.

Once Daniel and I had been apart for a while it was clear that the family home needed to be sold and we needed to each get our own place. I was determined to find a way to stay in the neighbourhood. With the changing living arrangements, I wanted to keep other things in the girls' lives as stable as possible. Same bus route to school, same local shops, close to friends, close to everything they knew. Close to their dad. I didn't want them to have the constantly shifting here and there, packing and unpacking childhood I'd experienced.

I sat down and did the sums. We had a modest mortgage. Once that was cleared, even if we got a great price for the family home, I'd walk away with less than half of what I'd need to buy a house in the area. A bank would never lend me the money I'd need on top of the deposit to get there.

I thought about the Glebe house Daniel and I had lived in when Sofia was born, only one suburb away, which Mum owned in the inner city. Three bedrooms, close to public transport. I could afford to pay what her tenants were paying at the time. I could stay there and provide a stable home for the girls while I worked out how the hell I was going to be able to buy a place in the neighbourhood they knew and loved.

It never occurred to me to ask Mum to help me hold on to the family home. But maybe she would have me as a tenant again?

I was scared to ask her. I called my sister. 'Do you think Mum might help me?' Maybe not me, but the girls? Sofia had just started high school and the twins had just started primary school. They were anxious and confused and sad, I could see it.

'I don't know,' is all Emily would say.

I didn't have the guts to call my mother and ask her over the phone, so I emailed.

'I need a place to stay close to our life in the inner west. Could I move back into the house in Glebe? I'll match whatever your tenants are paying. I don't want you to be out of pocket.'

I had to wait a few days for an answer. I couldn't sleep, could hardly eat.

It wasn't just that I was scared of Mum saying no and what that would mean for our relationship, which was already sketchy. I was churning all the time about how tenuous my living arrangements felt, my level of anxiety out of proportion with the reality of the situation. Some part of me felt as if I was back roaming the streets after a fight with my mother or sitting on the top of the covered part of the slippery dip wishing I'd packed a banana and more coins in my school case.

The roof above my head, the floor beneath my feet felt like they could be taken away from me at any time. And that felt worse because I was responsible for three children. It was also the roof above their heads and the floor beneath their feet.

My friends reassured me that it would be okay. 'She might not do it for you, but she'll think of her grandkids,' my friend Cecilia told me more than once.

And I told myself more than once, *I'm not asking for money. It's revenue neutral for her. I will pay her market rent. So maybe she will say yes.*

I thought, too, maybe she might remember what it was like to be mid-divorce, worried about money, responsible for children.

The email with my answer finally arrived. Short, sharp sentences. There would be no help. There were good tenants in the house. The next three months of my accommodation would be paid for. And finally, I should do better at saving then maybe I could afford to buy an apartment in the future.

The email had popped up while I was driving back to my apartment after dinner at a friend's house. I'd seen it, scanned it at the red light and then quickly turned into the closest street and parked so I could read it properly.

By a strange coincidence, I found myself parked outside the house in Glebe, the one I was hoping to rent.

I looked at the house. There were no lights on that I could see. Perhaps the reliable tenants were out; it was a Saturday night, after all. The garden Daniel and I had planted at the front was gone. Had it died or been pulled out? The house looked mostly the same, except a neat freak like me would never have a pile of shoes cluttering the doorstep.

It was when I was living there that things had really started to deteriorate with Mum, what with Sofia's birth and the stillbirth and everything else. I thought about Sofia on the toilet with her sapphire drop earrings and the Easter birthday party.

Was it right to say that was when things had started to fall apart? Maybe I just started to see it more clearly then, how disconnected, alienated, at odds Mum and I had always been.

I called my sister and told her about the email.

She said all the right, comforting words, and then she said something I'd never heard her say before.

'I'm calling Dad.'

*

Somewhere after divorce number two and in the middle of marriage number three, Dad created a discretionary trust for all his children. He emailed me about it at the time. The only thing I remember about the email is that it said the trust would dissolve when his youngest child turned twenty-one. Given he had a two-year-old son when the trust was created, I promptly put it out of my mind.

After Mum's email about the Glebe house, Emily called Dad like she'd promised. She told him about my situation and asked if there was any way to extract my share of the trust, given that I needed it now, not decades into the future.

To his credit, Dad agreed straight away. I thanked Emily for doing what I didn't have the stomach to do anymore: ask my parents for help.

Discretionary trusts are funny things. They are extremely useful if you aren't exactly sure how you want to distribute your estate. You basically pass the decision over to a trustee or trustees. As named beneficiaries of the trust, Emily and I had no rights. We didn't even have the right to have our questions about the trust answered. I was in the hands of the two men Dad had named as the trustees, one of his brothers and a family friend.

They were professional and conscientious men. They told us trusts couldn't just be wound up quickly like a bank account. It would take a few months for the trust to be sorted. Six months, probably. I was unfazed. I could wait.

*

After cycling in and out of the family home since we'd separated, it was time to sell and transition the girls to one week on and one week off in different houses.

During his off weeks, Daniel had been living with his sister. He moved into the family home permanently while we prepared to sell it. My tiny apartment wasn't big enough for four, so I rented a house in the street parallel to the family home. I was still determined to try to keep life as familiar as possible for the girls.

From the back bedroom window of this two-storey fibro house, you could see the red roof of the family home. When the twins were sad and missing their father, I'd hug them and say, 'We can go wave to him now, would you like that? Should we walk over to see him? We don't even need to put our shoes on.'

As I walked up to the door of my new digs, freshly cut keys in my hand, ready to start unpacking, my new neighbour burst out of her front door.

'Do you have children?' she barked at me.

She looked well over sixty, with a permanently disgruntled face, and dirty blonde hair in cropped waves close to her head.

'Yes, I do. My name's Rebecca, by the way.'

'Well, you better make sure there's carpet in your hallway for when they're running up and down or I'll be able to hear them when I'm watching TV.'

'Okay, I'll do that. I didn't catch your name.'

'It's Jan,' she mumbled over her shoulder as she headed back inside, slamming the flyscreen door behind her.

That day I went out and ordered carpet for all the rooms downstairs, including an extra-thick one for the hallway.

The first week the girls moved into the house with me, I took them over to introduce them to Jan.

'I've told the girls to be mindful when they're running in the house, and I've ordered carpet. It's arriving this week.'

Jan grunted 'Good', then off she went without a goodbye, slamming the flyscreen door.

After that, Jan and her less-outspoken husband would mostly ignore me, but I would sometimes get a half-decent hello from her when I saw her in the street.

This rented house was well positioned, but after a few weeks I realised what a total shit-box it really was. No effective air-conditioning. No insulation. We froze in winter, but at least we could fire up portable oil heaters and invest in more blankets. In summer, the heat was stifling. We had to keep to one room where the air-conditioning worked the best. The chocolate in the pantry melted into pools. When it rained, water trickled down the walls. The flyscreens were slashed, so when I opened the windows in the evening to get the hot air out, I'd let a squadron of bugs into the house.

I'd be on the phone to the agent all the time. *What about this? Can we fix this?* The answer was always no. To add insult to injury, along with eye-watering rents and house prices, Australian tenancy laws are some of the weakest in the Western world.

I was working like a demon at the time, six or seven days a week when the kids weren't staying with me. I had the cash to dip into my own pocket to fix the flyscreens and put a garden into the front and back yards, where before there had been only dirt and half-dead plants. I wanted the house to be beautiful and comfortable for the girls, and was willing to spend money to achieve that. But I couldn't do much about the heating and cooling.

'Is this our forever home?' Stella asked me one night as I was putting her to bed.

'God no,' I told her. 'My dad is going to give me some money, so I promise this time next year we will be in our own place.'

'Where?'

'Somewhere near here, I promise.'

*

I'd never raised with Mum the email rejecting my request to rent the Glebe house. She never spoke about it either. We spoke on the phone once a week. I'd visit her. She wasn't particularly interested in visiting me, but that was not unusual.

'Has Dad's money come yet?' That was always her first question when we'd talk.

'No, it's going to take a while, maybe six months tops.'

One sunny spring afternoon, we were entertaining our friends Louise and Tony and their twin girls. They'd come to visit our new puppy. The girls were running around the backyard with the dog while their parents chatted and drank coffee, then they took him out the front for a sniff and a wee.

Suddenly the kids all came running back into the house.

'The next-door neighbour yelled at us. She said we were laughing too loudly. She told us to shut up.'

Christ. Jan.

'Okay, maybe we should all go back inside,' I said.

The next day, as I was coming back from a trip to the shops, Jan was waiting for me out the front.

'Your children make a lot of noise.'

'I'm sorry about that, Jan. But you know I only have them fifty per cent of the time.'

She glared at me.

'I wish you didn't have them at all. I wish the police would come and take them away from you.'

Before I could respond, she scurried into her house and slammed the screen door.

A few weeks later, Dad died.

And as we tried to get his memorial together, a second, harsher lockdown loomed, and we were forced to cancel it.

As Sydney prepared for lockdown and I contemplated homeschooling my children next door to Jan, I got a call from my doctor. I'd had some elective surgery booked for later in the year.

'It's do it now or you'll have to wait for another year or so,' he told me. The hospitals were cancelling elective surgery, getting ready for the next wave of COVID admissions.

I decided to get the procedure done the next day.

Strangely enough, the thought of a hospital stay seemed like a holiday. A really deep sleep, food brought to me on a tray. I could watch TV without interruption. A staycation with Endone.

I admitted myself to an almost empty ward. The procedure went well. I woke up in a clean and comfortable room on my own. I hadn't been under a general anaesthetic for decades. I felt good – woozy, but good. After a few minutes my nurse bustled in, a friendly, diminutive woman.

'We need to get you to urinate to make sure your kidneys are working. I'll bring the bedpan over so you don't have to move.'

'It's fine. I can walk.'

'Do you need help? I can help you.'

'No, it's fine. I can do it myself.'

I remember shuffling to the bathroom and sitting on the toilet thinking it might be nice to have a cup of tea when I went back to bed.

The next thing I knew, I was on the cold floor. I could feel a man's body behind me, holding me, and my robe crumpled up around my waist. I realised my small hospital bathroom was crammed full of people. I opened my eyes to see about eight people looking at me. I felt mounting pain on the left side of my face, getting worse by the second.

'Hey, hey darling. Can you hear me?' The man in front of me was staring at me intently. 'What's your name?'

'My name's Rebecca.'

'Okay, good. Who is the Prime Minister of Australia? Do you know? Can you tell me who the Prime Minister is?'

'That motherfucker.'

He laughed. 'You need to be more specific.'

'Scott Morrison.'

'I think she's okay.'

I'd passed out due to a drop in blood pressure and fallen over face first. I banged my head, and my glasses cut my eye. I'd been out for a few minutes – my nurse had raised the alarm. I needed a brain scan, and they kept me in for an extra day for observation.

I still looked a fright when I returned home. The girls were dismayed. I'd come out with a rejuvenated urethra but I looked like I'd been the loser in a cat fight at an old-school pub.

The four of us and Shadow the puppy settled in for the night. I suggested we watch a comedy – we all needed a laugh. And we laughed a lot, sitting together, the twins with their legs draped over me, the puppy curled up in his bed at our feet. I was sore, but happy.

Halfway through the film I thought I could hear noises in the garden. Cats sometimes found their way into my newly planted shrubs. As I stood up to shoo them away I heard a thumping, a banging sound, like someone was hitting the side of the house with a bat.

I went out the front. There were plants lying scattered in my garden, pulled out by their roots. This wasn't cats. I heard Jan's screen door slam.

I went back inside and told the girls to stay put.

As I started to think about my next move, I saw the motion sensor light on our back porch turn on.

Our house was less than a metre away from Jan's house. If we were so inclined, from our respective porches we could reach out and stroke each other's cheeks with ease.

Mercifully, she and her husband didn't spend much time outside.

I walked towards the back of the house and opened the sliding door, but before I stepped out onto the porch, I could hear her. Breathing heavily, erratically. Jan was just standing there, so close to my back door that the sensor light had turned on. So close it was like she was breathing down my neck.

'Jan, if you continue to behave this way, I will call the police. You need to leave me and my children alone. Go back inside now.'

I closed the sliding door.

We had to leave. Before lockdown, before homeschooling started. Before she really lost her mind, and before I lost mine.

I called the real estate agent, told them the story. They didn't seem surprised.

'She's a character, Jan. Other tenants have had problems.'

I had to file a police report in order to break my lease. Without it, I'd have to pay out the lease, which didn't run out for another two months.

Two policemen arrived the next day. One very young, the other a little older.

They apologised for taking so long to respond and I apologised for wasting their time. I didn't need them to talk to Jan or do anything. I just needed to report her behaviour so I could break my lease without losing thousands of dollars.

The older policeman had a good look at my shiner.

'Oh, this,' I said jauntily. 'I was in hospital a few days ago and passed out. It's not domestic violence or anything.'

'I would have had to ask about it,' he said. Apparently, with a second lockdown on its way, they spent their days going from one domestic conflict to the next, households falling apart, neighbours at each other over the fence.

'People are losing it,' he told me.

*

I had to find a new place, and fast. There wasn't a lot on the market in the area that suited a family of four and would accept a dog. I was lucky to get a nice place in the next suburb, walking distance from Sofia's high school.

The agent asked me if I wanted a six-month lease or twelve months. I had no idea.

I had thought by then I'd be in a place of my own, bought with the money from the trust. It had been over a year since Dad had told me he'd dissolve it. Since then, we'd had no news. Any tentative requests for more information had yielded very little. The trustees said they were under no legal obligation to tell me anything. The lawyers my sister and I consulted told us the same thing.

I called my mother to tell her I was moving and to explain what had happened with Jan.

'When is the money arriving from the trust?' she asked me for the hundredth time.

'I told you, I don't know. I'm not allowed to know. I have no power over this process. It could be months. It could be years. No-one will tell me anything.'

Feeling hopeful, I opted for a six-month lease.

We moved in and on the first night the kids spent in the new place, Stella asked me again, 'Is this our forever home?'

'No, it isn't. I'm sorry. I know I said the next time we moved it would be into our forever home. I'm trying.'

Just before Christmas that year, about eight weeks after we'd moved, I was walking the puppy in the park. I stumbled across a family walking their poodle cross, and as I watched our dogs do the usual bum-sniffing routine, I realised that the kids looked familiar. The mum and I exchanged smiles.

'Our kids are in the same year at school,' she said.

We chatted about class sizes and teachers and homeschooling.

'Weren't we living in the same street for a while?' she asked, like she already knew the answer.

'I was, yes.'

Turns out this woman had lived in the same street until she upsized to a better place on the other side of the suburb.

'You were living next to Jan?'

'Yes. She was the main reason I had to leave. She was hostile and I didn't feel safe there anymore.'

'We got to know her a bit. She's not a bad sort of person. She's had a hard life. Her husband is really unwell. She was one of a group of women who were the first to try IVF in the 1970s. She tried and tried to have kids, but it never happened. I don't think she ever really recovered.'

Despite the ruined garden and the banging on the side of the house and the pain in the arse she'd been from the moment I arrived to the moment I left, I felt a surge of compassion for Jan.

It reminded me we are, all of us, recovering from something.

*

By Christmas 2021, as the lockdowns started to ease, I began to contemplate my next move. So much had happened between the end of the first lockdown and the end of the second. I was officially divorced, the financial arrangements finalised and the family home sold. The girls were now into the swing of moving from house to house. I could imagine all this might feel normal soon enough.

And yet I would lie in bed each night wondering what to do, how to get some certainty and security in my living arrangements. My six-month lease had passed and I had been offered a month-by-month lease. That meant if the trust money arrived, I could leave within a month without financial penalty. It also meant I could be given four weeks' notice to vacate, and have to move yet again.

Should I just bite the bullet, take the money I had and buy a place an hour or so away from where we were now? Or should I keep waiting?

Emily had been my great supporter through all this. The divorce, the constant moving and all the opaque dealings about the trust. That whole period of my life might have been intolerable without her. It might have broken me.

One November morning, as I was sitting in the backyard with a coffee and the dog, Emily called me. Mum had been repeatedly asking her about the trust. She'd explained that the trust could be tied up for years.

'I told Mum you need help now and we need to help you now. We can't rely on this money turning up anytime soon.'

'I don't think that's a good idea,' I replied. 'She was pretty clear about not helping me financially. She wouldn't even let me move into Glebe and pay market rent.'

Emily assured me that Mum was willing. She'd sell an apartment she owned near Bronte beach and give me a chunk of change from the proceeds.

I resisted the idea for a couple of weeks. I didn't want her to sell any property to help me. But Mum kept insisting. She wanted to do this for me, she said.

'What's all this property for anyhow?' she'd say playfully during our phone calls. 'For you and the girls.'

'But what if you sell and give me the money and then the trust money arrives?' I'd ask.

'Keep both.'

And so it was agreed, and yet the knot in my stomach remained. It all felt familiar. The offer of help extended. Then the backsliding, and the anger and resentment on both sides. But perhaps this time would be different. Perhaps all the moving and the incident with Jan and the impact on the children, and the uncertainty with the trust had helped change her mind.

I applied for a loan. The bank required Mum to sign an affidavit stating that a property she owned outright would be sold in February 2022 and a nominated amount from the sale of that property would be given to me.

'Do you really think she will go ahead?' I'd ring my sister every time the knot tightened.

'She's not going to go back on her word. You have it in writing. She signed an affidavit.'

I would look at that affidavit every few days. It was very clear about her intentions.

When the girls asked when we were moving again, I told them, 'Dad's money is taking some time, but Nonna will help.'

Christmas passed, then it was nearly the end of January. February was coming. I was scared to ask. Scared to raise it.

It was the bank that triggered the discussion. 'Are you ready to sign the mortgage paperwork now that the investment property is sold?'

Again, I didn't call Mum. I didn't even email. Yet again, I called my sister. 'How are the plans for the sale of the apartment going?'

'I don't know,' she said.

So, I called my mother and got the answering machine. 'Just asking about the sale of the property, how's it going?'

She didn't call back, but I got an email from her partner saying he'd respond the next day.

The email arrived in language so devoid of emotion, so formal, it was as if he was writing to a stranger, not someone he'd known for forty years. Like he was sending an email to an unreliable tenant about a breach of their tenancy agreement.

The apartment would not be sold, as a sale would trigger a large amount of capital gains tax and this would, ideally, be avoided.

If in six months the trust money didn't arrive, they would find a way to help me. He wanted to make it very clear that this would compromise their financial future but nevertheless, they were prepared to do that.

The knot turned into that sinking feeling, so familiar and yet shocking all the same.

I called my sister, sobbing.

'It's not the money. I didn't ask for the money. She offered. It's the way they treat me. It's the raising my hopes and then the disappointment.'

Stupidly, I tried to call my mother. I knew she was at home but she let the call go to the machine. I screamed and raged down the phone. Emily tried to talk to my mother but she kept hanging up on her.

I sent them another email.

What you do with your money is your business.
I understand why you made the decision you did, not to sell because you didn't want to pay tax. It's the way you communicate with me. Can we sit down together and talk about how we communicate?

For two days, there was silence.

Then on the third day, I received a long email from Mum's partner.

This was, in itself, a notable event. I'd known him since I was ten. Mum had met him through work, when they were both teachers in the Catholic school system. He had joined the Christian Brothers out of high school. In his early fifties he left the order, moved into my old bedroom and never moved out.

He and I weren't close. He was a self-contained man, and I was grateful to him because he was my mother's dedicated companion. He did almost everything for her around the house, and managed and maintained all the rental properties. He fetched shopping and emptied kitty litter. He travelled with her on cruises and drove her around and put the bins out on collection day. He had been her main carer throughout the first cancer and the second.

I can't recall once in the forty years I'd known him ever having a meaningful conversation with him. And in recent years exchanging anything more than a hello and goodbye on the phone. In my late twenties, I complained to Mum about how shallow our relationship was, this man I'd known almost my whole life, who was practically her husband.

'Why do you want a relationship with him? What a waste of time.'

Anyhow, after four decades it seemed that he felt sufficiently moved to say something more than hello and goodbye to me. To write a two-page email, no less.

It was all there in black and white. Things my mother had said about me over the years in an email from her partner. It detailed what I knew she thought of me. She'd said versions of the things in the email to my face, and I'd been told that she expressed these opinions to my sister, my friends, and to Daniel's family when he and I were married.

The email stated directly that my mother hadn't broken a promise.

That helping me would risk their financial future.

That the commitment to help was only if Dad's money was never going to arrive. That my plan was to collect money from my mother and my father.

That my comments that my mother was always letting me down were 'pathetic'.

That my behaviour towards my mother was appalling, insulting.

That she was the most loving and attentive parent, looking after me for over fifty years.

That I had been self-centred in all of my relationships; that I believe I am always the victim and everybody else is to blame.

That I walk around with the attitude that 'Poor Rebecca doesn't deserve this.'

That I switch from Charm Offensive to Emotional Vitriol within seconds if I don't get what I want.

He ended it by saying he hoped I would not go off in yet another rage after reading the email.

There it was. I was lucky, really, to have it there in black and white, instead of the depth of his and my mother's resentment towards me revealing itself in bewildering flashes over the years.

I thought back to the time I dropped the flowers off while she was lying in bed in the darkness.

'Whenever you come to see me, you bring nice things ... I always think, I wonder what Rebecca wants from me now?'

There was the gut punch of reading the email. The shock. And then the turning inward. *Is any of this true? Am I this person? Maybe I am. Maybe they are right.*

Then the anger. *That's not true. I need to see them and tell them this isn't true, convince them of my true nature and good intentions.*

All of this took less than a minute to wash through me – the shock, the self-doubt, the anger, the determination to put things right.

And then there was something new, at least when it came to my mother. Not unlike the feeling I'd had in the law school basement with my father.

It felt like letting go. Forgiveness. No, more like acceptance.

It's funny, when you reach breaking point with a person it actually feels like a 'break', a movement inside your body, in your chest or in your gut. Like when you're bending a tree branch and you keep bending and bending it until it snaps into two, the edges all fresh wood, sap and splinters.

That's what I felt once I'd ridden the flash wave of shock, self-doubt, anger and self-righteousness.

The snap.

I was done. I called my sister.

'I think it's best if you don't see Mum anymore,' she said. Having her blessing was important. In the past when Mum and I had fought and been estranged, I'd been scared of losing Emily as well. But not now.

I put the phone down and sent an email back in response.

It was short, and I found the right words, a rare thing at such a stressful moment.

> *If you are right about who I am, then I wouldn't want a person like that in your life. If you are wrong about me, then I can't have people in my life who think this way about me.*

I told them they had access to the children whenever they wanted through Emily. I told them to take care, and look after themselves.

This exchange of emails and the call to Emily, took less than an hour.

I've read and re-read that back and forth, his original email and my response, over and over. Just to see if I remember the contents accurately. If I still believe I did the right thing.

I do. I did. I had a clear choice between a relationship with my mother and my own peace of mind.

I chose myself.

And she made the same choice.

After that email, I never heard from my mother again.

The MDMA helped me understand everything that happened leading up to that moment with greater clarity. It wasn't that Mum didn't want to help me and her grandchildren in theory. But when she had to follow through, she couldn't. Perhaps her wealth, the houses she owned, keeping all that close and in her control, that's what made her feel safe and secure after so many years of abuse by my father.

And it felt like this mattered to her more than anything else.

*

It's hard to tell you this story, and not just because it's still painful to relive it. It's because in telling it, I worry I sound like Veruca Salt in *Charlie and the Chocolate Factory.*

'I want my trust fund money nooowwwww Daddy!'

You shouldn't feel sorry for me. It all worked out in the end. I'm lucky, and I rarely lose sight of that. I've had my fair share of trauma but I've also had my fair share of oxygen facials and grazing tables. I'm doing okay.

I was trying my best to feel lucky when I called the bank after the email exchange with mum's partner.

'The money isn't coming from the sale of the apartment.'

'What about the trust money?' he asked me.

'No idea.'

'Well, we're going to have to start from scratch when it comes to the loan.'

I told him I'd be in touch when things changed.

I didn't have the heart to tell the girls that our forever home was getting further and further away from me.

I started to hatch a plan. No-one was going to swoop in and save me. I had a decent deposit. A good income. I'd just have to look outside the neighbourhood, down the train line – away from everything the girls knew, yes, but we had each other. They'd adjust and I'd forgive myself at some stage for making promises that I couldn't keep.

That was February 2022. By mid-year lockdown was well and truly over, and life in Sydney was returning to normal. In late June, I talked my friends Sarah and Amy into coming on a day trip to the wineries in the Hunter Valley.

Throughout my life, Mum always warned me about being too close to people who weren't family.

After friends had come over to visit me or when I'd finish a long phone call with one of them, she'd pull me aside and say, 'It's nice you've got friends but don't get too invested in them. You can't really trust them, you can only trust family.'

One of the many pieces of advice over the years dished out by my mother that I mostly ignored. Friends had supported me through every one of life's challenges. Sarah and Amy had been two people who had been particularly loving since my marriage ended.

I decided the three of us deserved a trip to the country, lunch and ridiculous chitchat with cellar door staff about soil quality and tannins.

We made it out of Sydney traffic easily and were at least an hour early for our lunch reservation. We decided to take a quick detour to a new winery down the road from the restaurant I'd booked. We were the first and only people that early at the cellar door. The manager, who was also the wine maker, led us out onto the terrace and sat us at a little table.

It was a cool, windless and sunny winter's day. There were a few clouds above, and an uninterrupted view of the vines in front of us.

If this is life, it's good, I thought. *I'm happy, I'm healthy. So are the girls. I have a job. A chunk of change in the bank. I have Emily, my friends. This is enough. I can make this work.*

My phone buzzed. I picked it up. An email from my uncle, the trustee. I hadn't heard from him in months, not since Christmas the year before.

The trust was resolved. The money would be deposited the following week. More than I expected. More than enough for that forever home in the neighbourhood we called home.

I looked up.

'The trust money is coming,' I told my friends.

Before they had the chance to say anything in response the winemaker had arrived with three champagne flutes and an open bottle.

'Shall we start with a glass of sparkling wine?'

'Yes,' yelled Sarah. 'And fill them up to the brim.'

Inheritance

In her extensively researched and compelling book *I Feel Love: MDMA and the Quest for Connection in a Fractured World*, *New York Times* journalist Rachel Nuwer writes about how MDMA enthusiasts believe that the drug can play a central role in a mass mental health movement 'in the service of world peace'.[28]

She writes that these men and women committed to the use of MDMA as a therapeutic tool argue that it can do more than help individuals and couples. They believe the drug can reveal a vision of 'a different kind of future, one in which love, empathy, and unity were paramount'.[29]

Once upon a time, before I'd done the MDMA therapy, I would have rolled my eyes at such a suggestion. Let's face it, without having done the therapy, I would never have read Nuwer's book in the first place. But if my experience is any guide, this drug holds potential beyond its use to treat complex trauma. If we nail the right ways to introduce it to the public, it could play a part in addressing complex social problems.

There is no doubt that the MDMA therapy helped me unlock my own capacity for self-healing.

The magic of MDMA, from my perspective, is that it helps us forge connections. In describing its impact to friends, I said it was like watching the pieces of a shattered mirror slowly and surely reassemble themselves into a whole, like a scene in a Harry Potter film. Trauma shatters your sense of self; you repress or twist memories into shapes to make them more tolerable. The MDMA helps reassemble that broken picture. The cracks are still there, but you can see yourself in a new, more integrated way.

I could understand, and more importantly *feel*, how my lifelong sense of insecurity, of feeling unsafe, stretched back in time to my mother and my grandmother. Probably back further, to women in my family whose names I'll never know. And that all my best and worst behaviour was driven by this desire to feel safe. If I've achieved anything as a mother, I think it's that I've given my children a sense of safety and security that I never experienced.

I wish I could say the MDMA therapy 'cured me'. Memoirs like this are supposed to end with some kind of comforting resolution. I'm happy now. I've arrived, forgiven, evolved.

But it's not that simple. I struggle still with self-compassion. I grasp it for a few moments and then it melts away. At least I am letting myself grasp for it. I still clean like a maniac. Get overwhelmed and get angry. But I can stand back and observe myself overreacting, spiralling and know why. The whirligig still turns, worse on some days than others. But in so many other ways, I am calmer. I let myself relax more. I push myself less.

Gabor Maté writes that 'we are never as close as we hope or as far as we fear'.[30] He's right.

When I am walking the dogs or lying in bed at night or chopping up vegetables in my kitchen and I feel overwhelmed by resentment, at the cruelty and manipulation and indifference of my parents, I close my eyes. I breathe in and out. And I go back to the feeling of my mother sitting by my sick bed, her look of concern and the cool flannel on my head. I go back to what it felt like to hold Sofia for the first time. To look out across the Byron hinterland towards the Pacific Ocean and feel part of that glorious expanse of nature.

I think too about what MDMA therapy has taught me, not just about trauma and its impacts, but about the social systems that not only inflict trauma but thrive on it.

MDMA has given me a whole new, visceral understanding of the connections between the human world and the natural world. As an environmentalist, it's deepened my commitment to acting on climate change. It's given me new insight into the flaws in the way we approach mental health: reactive, dominated by the interests of pharmaceutical companies more concerned with repeat prescriptions than healing, and in ways that aren't even helping the wealthiest of us, let alone those living with poverty, racism and displacement.

MDMA therapy was possible for me because I had the resources, money, time and social support to access it. Especially given it was illegal. It was safer and more effective because of the decades of talk therapy I'd been able to afford. It worked because, trauma aside, I was otherwise healthy, physically safe and financially secure. I was unravelling while in a position of privilege that my race, class and nationality provide.

Terms like 'intergenerational trauma' and 'social determinants of health' are words I've read and said so many times, but before MDMA I can honestly say I didn't have a sliver of understanding of what I was talking about.

What would it be like to undergo MDMA therapy facing issues of intergenerational trauma in the context of colonialism, slavery, homophobia? With little hope of ever feeling safe in your own home, your neighbourhood, the country you live in?

I thought about this every day after my first session, as I felt the full weight of all I'd experienced in a world which, on the whole, was a welcoming, rather than hostile, place for me.

But of all the gifts that the MDMA therapy bestowed on me, the most important was empathy.

It helped me understand my parents and what I'd inherited from them.

The good and the bad.

*

Angus and Maureen were close family friends of my parents when I was growing up. They were an older couple but more like kind elder siblings than parental figures. Their friendship with my parents pre-dated my birth and I can't quite remember how they met. It was Adelaide in the 1960s, so perhaps within certain circles everyone ended up knowing everyone else.

They lived in a stylish modern house in the Adelaide Hills. Angus was an interior designer, lean and bald with a beard, impeccably dressed. Effusive. We would arrive at their home for a weekend lunch and he would greet us the same way every time. Wide smile, arms outstretched, barrelling towards us, laugh-shouting, 'Hello, hello, hello.' He seemed delighted to see us in a way no-one other than my nonna ever seemed delighted to see us.

Maureen was much quieter than her husband and seemed, to my childish eyes, like an angel. She had this gentle quality, dreamy brown eyes in a round face framed by a cap of curly brown hair. She represented a different kind of welcome than her husband, a soft landing in a home that felt safer than my own.

Their sprawling house was full of exotic objects they seemed happy for me to pick up and examine. On one visit, I saw a small grasshopper made from straw and paper on a bookshelf.

'Pick it up, Rebecca,' Maureen told me. 'But remember it's fragile.' I told her I didn't know what fragile meant, and she explained it to me. 'Fragile means easy to break if you aren't careful.'

Another time, I saw what looked like a bumpy red apple in a bowl in their kitchen. Angus took a knife and carved open the mysterious fruit for me. It was a pomegranate. I'd had no idea something that exotic existed in the same category as pears and bananas. He sat me down in a leather chair in the lounge room and showed me how to carefully pick out the seeds one by one and eat them. He told me it was mine and I slowly, joyously ate the whole thing.

Years later, when I was an adult, Angus gave me a box of letters my parents had sent to him and Maureen during the first few years after I was born, when they were living in Oxford.

I had leafed through the contents when Angus first gave them to me without paying much attention to the detail.

By then Dad was sick, but still alive. I was still doing what I could to get close to Mum.

I put the box into a much larger one where I kept all my nostalgic bumf, newspaper clippings and old photos and the bits and pieces of lace handmade by my nonna.

A few weeks after my final MDMA session, I pulled the box out, ready to carefully read through all the letters. I decided to make myself a strong drink and ignite the fire pit in the courtyard of my house. These letters, I thought, would be full of the early warning signs of what was to come. I would read, reflect and burn.

Once the fire was self-sustaining, I sat cross-legged on the padded garden lounge and opened the box. There was a good-sized bundle, letters written with blue fountain pen on thin, pale blue paper with almost undetectable blue lines. Some were on small, now brittle pieces of white paper. And a few were on those postcard-sized aerogrammes that folded out, my father's script shrinking to an almost indecipherable size in order to cram as many words as possible onto the fine paper.

Dad wrote more letters than Mum. My father's script was neat, elegant and contained. My mother's was less legible, and with more dramatic swoops of the pen, the y's reaching down to touch the tips of the letters on the lines below.

The letters started and ended with 'We miss you', 'We can't wait to see you', 'Thank you for your generous gift, your last letter'. Dad's letters were full of reflections about politics in Britain and Australia. Mum's were about the cold weather she hated so much and the British people, who she also wasn't fond of. Counting the weeks and months before they could visit Italy.

Once I was born, my father's letters read like any letter from a young father, full of stories of first steps and first colds, vaccinations and feeding the ducks at the park. Mum wrote about these events as well, in fewer words. She was busier, I expect, actually dealing with the first steps and the first colds and stopping me from falling into the pond with the ducks.

And there was so much affection. For each other and for me. In every single letter.

In one letter Dad calls me 'la bimba' – Italian for 'baby girl' – and laments that I won't be able to spend time with Mum's parents at any point soon so won't be learning to speak some Italian.

He expresses his concerns about finishing his PhD in time, about having enough money and being able to get a job when he returns to Australia. He then brushes these worries away like crumbs off a table. 'There is so much happiness in things too.'

It's my mother's letters that I spend the most time with. A few weeks after my birth, she writes, 'A short note from a very happy mum. Rebecca Jane is just so beautiful. I can't believe she is ours and I keep having to remind myself she is real. She looks so much like [her dad]. Turned up nose, blue eyes and masses of black hair.'

She signs off another short letter with these words: 'Today, finally a warm lovely day and so I shall close with a final description. [Dad] on chair, reading poetry, [me] beside him writing, baby in carry-cot sleeping, all in the most beautiful English garden in the afternoon.'

Underneath the letters, two handmade books of poetry and stories they had created together for me. Words by Dad, illustrations by Mum. Poems about hedgehogs and giraffes and ducks that dance and some made-up creature called a Poogle.

And then at the bottom of all this paper, a photo I'd never seen. One of the letters had mentioned a photo enclosed, the first portrait of the three of us.

Dad looks so young because he was, he was only twenty-three. A mess of black hair, gold-rimmed glasses and a five-o'clock shadow. He looks every bit the post-grad. Mum with her long, straight dark hair, parted in the middle, wearing a dress I vaguely remember, white with a Florentine flower pattern in orange and brown.

And me, only a few months old, in an orange jumper, looking exactly like my mother had described in the letter. Masses of dark hair, turned-up nose, shiny beady eyes.

Dad is holding onto me with two hands, his fingers grasped around my tummy, and in my clenched little fist are my mother's fingers.

They are fresh-faced and beautiful and smiling like they are happy, full of hope and good intentions.

No-one has children in order to fuck them up.

I put the faded papers – the letters and the poems – back in the box and watched the fire burn to coals.

I kept the photo out. I thought hard about the good. That's what trauma does. When you block out the bad, it can rob you of the good.

I remembered a time Dad took Emily and me into town in the early hours of the morning for pancakes in our pyjamas. About AA Milne and walks to the sea and gelato.

But mostly, I tried to focus on Mum, and on one memory that I keep coming back to.

When I was ten, I picked up George Orwell's *Animal Farm* from our bookcase. Both my parents encouraged me to read it. I thought it would be about animals. And at some level, it was.

Boxer the horse was my favourite character and when he died, I was distraught.

I rushed to my mother's bedroom after finishing the book and threw myself into her arms.

'Boxer dies. They killed him and pretended they didn't.'

'I know.'

'I'm going to die one day too. What's going to happen when I die?'

My mother looked at me with such seriousness and compassion. She gave me the best, most honest, most loving answer I can recall her ever giving to a question I asked her.

'I don't know. No-one really knows. I just can't imagine that when I die, the love I have for you won't keep on living.'

Needless to say, I didn't burn the papers or the poems that day or any other day.

I keep the photo of my parents with a photo of my sister, a small piece of pale pink lace handmade by my nonna and three little worry dolls, tiny girls with red bows in their hair, that I bought from the market the day I moved into our forever home.

I keep them in a box made from sassafras wood, to remind me of the only things worth protecting in this world shaped as much by love as it is by loss.

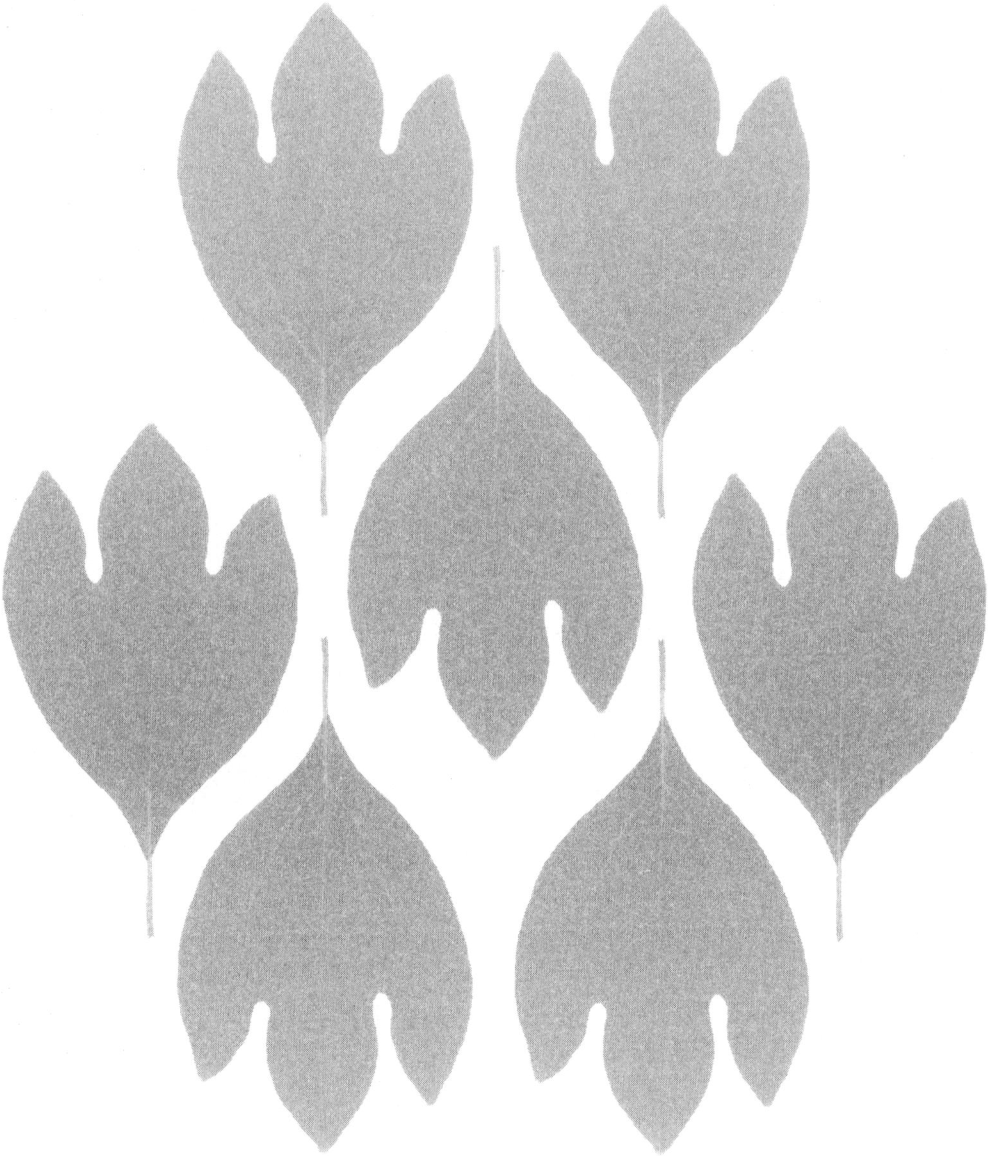

ACKNOWLEDGEMENTS

Thanks to friends who read early drafts and supported me throughout these last few years and through this process: Alex, Amy, Cecilia, Cisca, Clare, Daisy, Dan, Deanne, Dorothy, Felicity, Gillian, Hans, Helen, Holly, Ilona, James B, James J, James R, Jules, Kate, Linda, Lisa, Louise, Meredith, Mette, Michael, Moksha, Nicky, Sabina, Sarah, Sue, Suzie, Teya, Verity and Zoe. The rest of the Rosies and The Melbourne Girl Gang, thanks to you as well.

I am profoundly grateful to 'Abby'. To 'Karen'. And to my extraordinary children.

To my agent, Jeanne Ryckmans, and Key People Literary Management.

To Sophie Hamley, Jacquie Brown and Vanessa Lanaway and everyone from Hachette.

Written on the lands of the Wangal people of the Eora nation.

ENDNOTES

1 M Karr, *The Art of Memoir*, HarperCollins, New York, 2015, p. 11.

2 ibid, p. 32.

3 K Andrews, *Wanderers: A History of Women Walking*, Reaktion Books, London, 2020, p. 38.

4 O Winfrey and B Perry, *What Happened to You? Conversations on Trauma, Resilience, and Healing*, Pan Macmillan, London, 2021, p. 28.

5 Jill Norman (ed), *Elizabeth David's Christmas*, Michael Joseph, London, 2003, p. 11.

6 My process with Julia was inexpensive in comparison to the costs currently being discussed for MDMA treatment. For example, the MDMA therapy approved by the Australian government at this moment in time requires the supervision of two psychotherapists and could run to $25,000 out of pocket.

7 T Passie, 'The early use of MDMA ("Ecstasy") in psychotherapy (1977–1985)', *Drug Science, Policy and Law*, 2018, vol. 4.

8 R Riederer, 'The rebranding of MDMA', *The New Yorker*, 13 July 2023, newyorker.com.

9 In a setback for advocates of MDMA treatment, in early June 2024 the US Federal Drug Agency rejected MDMA as a safe treatment for PTSD. time.com/6985929/fda-advisors-reject-mdma-ptsd-treatment/

10 A Blau and G Thompson, '"Serious concerns" over TGA's decision making on landmark psilocybin, MDMA ruling', ABC News, 18 March 2023, abc.net.au.

11 Thanks to Michael for pointing this out to me after reading an early draft.

12 It's important to note that regardless of the potential benefits of MDMA for helping people with complex trauma, it may not be an appropriate path to take for people with a history of addiction.

13 J Mitchell, M Bogenschutz, A Lilienstein et al, 'MDMA-assisted therapy for severe PTSD: a randomized, double-blind, placebo-controlled phase 3 study', *Nature Medicine*, vol. 27, no. 6, 2021.

14 A Mandal, 'Efficacy of SSRIs for depression', *News Medical Life Sciences*, 10 June 2023, news-medical.net; 'Depression treatment after unsatisfactory response to SSRIs when used as first-line therapy', Effective Health Care (EHC) Program, 15 June 2010, effectivehealthcare.ahrq.gov; T Blackburn, 'Depressive disorders: Treatment failures and poor prognosis over the last 50 years', *Pharmacology Research & Perspectives*, May 2019, vol. 7, no. 3.

15 Z Rizmal, 'Australians are taking antidepressants in record numbers and for longer than ever, but coming off them can be "frightening"', ABC News, 22 February 2022, abc.net.au.

16 World Population Review, 'Antidepressant use by country 2023', worldpopulationreview.com; SingleCare, 'Prescription drug statistics 2023', 29 November 2023, singlecare.com; N Diaz-Camal, JD Cardoso-Vera, H Islas-Flores et al., 'Consumption and ocurrence [sic] of antidepressants (SSRIs) in pre- and post-COVID-19 pandemic, their environmental impact and innovative removal methods: A review', *Science of the Total Environment*, 2022, vol. 829.

17 S Trachman, 'Why is there an increase in depression after COVID?', *Psychology Today*, 3 June 2022, psychologytoday.com.

18 J Mitchell, M Bogenschutz, A Lilienstein et al, 'MDMA-assisted therapy for severe PTSD: a randomized, double-blind, placebo-controlled phase 3 study', *Nat Med* 27, 1025–1033 (2021). doi.org/10.1038/s41591-021-01336-3, p. 1032.

19 On this point I would recommend James Davies' *Sedated: How Modern Capitalism Created Our Mental Health Crisis*, Atlantic Books, London, 2022.

20 S Sontag, *Illness as Metaphor and AIDS and its Metaphors*, Farrer, Straus & Giroux, New York, 1978.

21 G Maté, *The Myth of Normal: Trauma, Illness and Healing in a Toxic Culture*, Random House, London, 2022, pp. 140–41.

22 J Bradley, 'A trip to the doctor: A personal experience of how psychedelics are transforming mental health therapies', *The Monthly*, August 2021, themonthly.com.au.

23 S Chenery, 'The never-ending fallout of the northern rivers floods: "People are just worn down"', *The Guardian*, 20 February 2023, www.theguardian.com.

24 G Albrecht, G-M Sartore, L Connor et al, 'Solastalgia: The Distress Caused by Environmental Change', *Australasian Psychiatry*, 2007;15(1_suppl):S95–S98. doi:10.1080/10398560701701288.

25 R Nuwer, *I Feel Love: MDMA and the Quest for Connection in a Fractured World*, Bloomsbury, London, 2023, p. 219.

26 An enemy alien was defined under the law as anyone over the age of sixteen who 'possesses the nationality of a State at war with His Majesty'. The definition included naturalised British subjects who were originally from the Axis power countries regardless of how long they had lived in Australia.

27 Australian Military Forces – Northern Command, report dated 20 October 1941.

28 R Nuwer, *I Feel Love: MDMA and the Quest for Connection in a Fractured World*, Bloomsbury, London, 2023, p. 75.

29 ibid, p. 93.

30 G Maté, *The Myth of Normal: Trauma, Illness and Healing in a Toxic Culture*, Random House, London, 2022, p. 430.

If you would like to find out more about Hachette Australia, our authors, upcoming events and new releases you can visit our website or our social media channels:

hachette.com.au
HachetteAustralia
HachetteAus